# Stop Cancer in its Tracks:
# Your Path to Mindfulness in Healing Yourself

By Jerome Freedman, Ph. D.

Copyright (c) 1997, 2014 Jerome Freedman, Ph. D.
ALL RIGHTS RESERVED
ISBN-13: 978-1-64370-180-6

Disclaimer:

This material is copyright(c) 1997 - 2014, by Jerome Freedman, Ph. D. All Rights Reserved. This document is meant to be a description of the author's experience and he in no way takes responsibility for the accuracy or completeness of any medical knowledge. The author assumes no responsibility for choices made by any of the readers of this material.

The author is not a physician and makes no claims about the potential usefulness of the subject matter herein to have any medical benefit. Please check with your doctor if you find something interesting that you would like to try.

Revised on July 24, 2018

## TABLE OF CONTENTS

Table of Contents ..................................................................... 3

Preface to the 2014 Edition ..................................................... 5

Preface to the 2018 Edition ..................................................... 7

Seven Principles of Mindfulness in Healing ........................... 9

Introduction ............................................................................ 13

1 - Onset of Disease ............................................................... 17

2 - Treatment Options ........................................................... 23

3 - Making the Decision ........................................................ 33

4 - Treatment Preparations ................................................... 41

5 - Accelerated Growth ......................................................... 49

6 - Treatment Begins ............................................................. 61

7 - Waiting for a Complete Response ................................... 73

8 - Almost Normal Life .......................................................... 85

9 - The Big Question ............................................................ 101

10 - Consolidation Treatment ............................................. 115

11 - Riding the Bull Home ................................................... 135

12 – Where Do We Go From Here? .................................... 145

13 - My New Career ............................................................. 163

14 - Days with Thich Nhat Hanh ......................................... 171

15 - Additional Treatments ................................................. 179

**16 - A New Episode** ............................................................ 191

**Epilog** ........................................................................... 199

**Parting Words** ............................................................... 201

**About The Author** ......................................................... 203

**Dedication** .................................................................... 205

**Acknowledgements** ....................................................... 207

## PREFACE TO THE 2014 EDITION

This book was begun with the onset of bladder cancer in 1997. I maintained an on-line diary for many months and kept it up for as long as it benefited my readers.

I found writing the diary to be extremely beneficial. It allowed me to keep track of all the different forms of medical treatment I was receiving, both traditional and alternative.

Additionally, the response I got to the postings each day inspired me to keep going knowing that many people with cancer and other life threatening illnesses would benefit from learning about alternative possibilities for their medical care.

The main objectives I had in keeping track of virtually everything medical, emotional, psychological, and spiritual that happened to me was to document my efforts to **take charge of my own healing experience**.

Now all of this information is available and I am thrilled to share it with other people going through a rough time with their health. My aim is to inspire you to be actively involved in everything that happens once serious illness strikes.

In the original version on my website, there were links to the resources and protocols that I followed in my treatment. Since most of these resources are more than seventeen years old, I have left them out of this version. My plan is to have an additional book with these resources updated. You can find many of them on the web at http://mindfulnessinhealing.org.

Inside this book, you will find information about a large number of alternative treatments that I engaged in from January 25, 1997 on. The different alternative treatments were in addition to surgery, radiation, and chemotherapy.

Alternative medicine is also known as complementary, integrative, and adjunctive medicine, depending on who you listen to. For brevity, I'll most often use *alternative medicine* when referring to any one of these practices.

A partial list of the alternative practices that I employed includes
- Mindfulness practices (see _Meditation Practices_ – http://mountainsangha.org) including sitting meditation, walking meditation, and guided meditation
- Guided imagery, also known as guided visualization and other

names
- Support groups
- Acupuncture
- Chiropractic
- Hyperbaric oxygen healing
- Sessions with shamans and other types of faith healers
- Massage
- Feldenkrais
- Herbs and supplements from all over the world
- Movement and dance therapy
- Art therapy
- Tai chi, Qi gong
- Reiki
- Tennis
- Yoga

This version contains the ***Seven Principles of Mindfulness in Healing*** which evolved over many years of exposure to alternative medicine practices. They are also the subject of my next book by the same name. The book will expand on each of the seven principles and illustrate them with examples.

## PREFACE TO THE 2018 EDITION

Inspired by Anita Moorjani's *Dying to Be Me: My Journey from Cancer, to Near Death, to True Healing*, I decided to publish this diary to a wider audience. Many people have been inspired by my story since 1997 and I continue to consult with people about cancer, mindfulness and meditation.

A strange thing happened in late February and early March of this year. I stopped wanting food and nothing appealed to me. My appetite disappeared for many weeks and my stomach began to ache. On my first visit to Dr. Martin Rossman, MD on March 10, he found normal vital signs and no indication of infection. Two day later, my stomach was really hurting a lot, so I scheduled another appointment with Marty and he ordered blood work for this visit. The second visit in March never happened as I was called by my urological oncologist at UCSF (Dr. Maxwell Meng) and ordered to check into the emergency room at UCSF Parnassus Hospital. My creatinine was 8.5 – a very dangerous level.

When a stent in my right ureter failed to drain the volume of stored up urine in my kidneys, nephrostomy tubes were placed in both kidneys and they began draining. It took about a week before the creatinine began to lower and I was finally discharged from the hospital after ten days.

In the meantime, my whole digestive system got stuffed up and I developed gastroparesis. This condition made it very difficult for me to eat normally and I suffered quite a bit. If I ate even on bite too much, my gastroesophageal sphincter would spasm and nothing could get in our out of my mouth. Over the months of March, April and May this difficulty persisted and finally began to lift with acupuncture with Marty, Chinese herbs from Marty and the relief of constipation. Now, thankfully, I am eating normally and enjoying food again!

I began immunotherapy treatments with Dr. Friedlander at UCSF on June 19. Keytrudy (pembrolizumab) has be cleared by the FDA for treatment of "advanced bladder cancer," so I'm covered for this expensive drug. So far, there have been no side effects and it seems to be working or Dr. Meng wouldn't even suggest capping the right nephrostomy tube.

So, here I am, 21 years later and still dealing with bladder cancer. This time, however, it is in the muscle layer and not visible during cystoscopy. It must be receding or Dr. Meng would insist on keeping the left nephrostomy tube as well as the right.

My attitude during these past six months of suffering and no tennis has been excellent. I have been resting a lot, writing little, and spending time with family and friends. Long walks have been quite refreshing and my energy is finally getting back to normal. By the time you read this paragraph, I should be playing tennis again. The key to my recovery lie in Mala's (my wife) unconditional love and caring, as well as her undying confidence that I would heal. Additional keys to my success include almost daily conversations with my daughters, visits from friends, and, of course, mindfulness practices.

I also recognized the importance of love. This was driven home not only by my kidney failure, but by a session of Theta Healing with Kimberly in Modesto and reading Anita Moorjani's book. It was the love of my wife, family and friends that helped me recover from kidney disease. It was Theta Healing that taught me more about unconditional love. And it was Anita Moorjani who inspired me in her Ted Talk in the Bay Area with these words:

> *I learned the most important thing we have here to focus our awareness on is love. That is number one and when I say love it's very easy to say or for us to say we need to love other people. But one of the things I learned is that one of the reasons I got cancer is because I didn't love myself! That's hugely important! When we love ourselves, we value ourselves. When we value ourselves, we teach people how to treat us. When you love yourself, you find no need to control or bully other people, nor do you allow other people to control or bully you. So loving yourself is as important as loving everybody else and the more you love yourself the more love you have to give other people.*

## SEVEN PRINCIPLES OF MINDFULNESS IN HEALING

The seven principles of Mindfulness in Healing are pervasive throughout the remaining chapters, if only implicitly. They have been part of my life since I began studying and practicing meditation and learning about natural healing. They probably date back to the time before my son had cancer in 1976 - see **Mind Stories Helped Cure Cancer** on *Meditation Practices*.

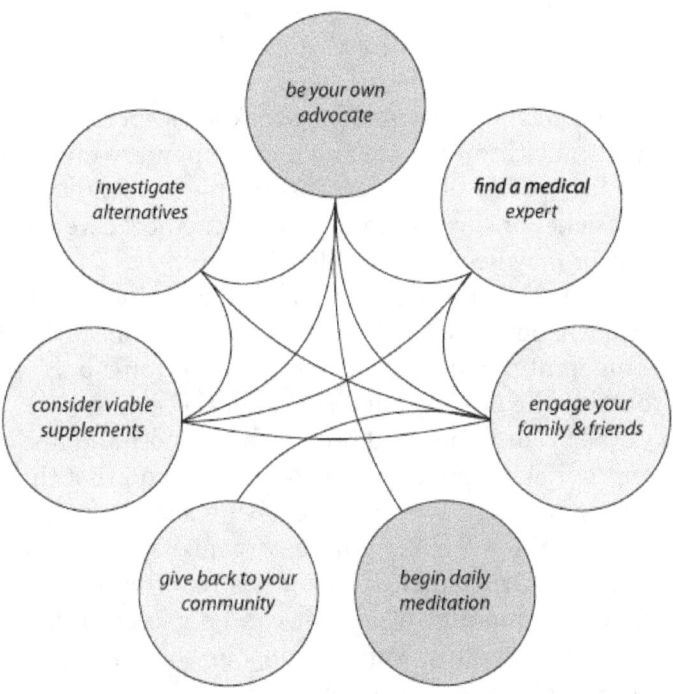

Seven Principles of Mindfulness in Healing

1. **Be an advocate for your own health care.** This means to take charge of your own health care and not leave everything up to the doctors. It is fine to listen to them and understand what they are asking you to do.

    However, you must take responsibility for your healing by being actively involved and being willing to explore possibilities. Getting second and third opinions may help.

    Talking to friends and relatives who are knowledgeable

about health matters can help.

Most of all, unless you have extreme circumstances, take a few days to think things over.

2. **Investigate alternatives and complementary healing methods to enhance your healing**. Many alternative treatments can relieve a lot of stress and suffering just by participating in them.

   To name a few, we have found that acupuncture, massage, Qi Gong, yoga and other movement therapies, meditation, and creative expression can really help.

   In participating in these kinds of activities, you are encouraged to do as much or as little as you feel comfortable doing.

3. Have a healing professional who knows about your standard medical treatment plan and complementary medicine to manage your well-being. Most people have only their primary physician or surgeon to rely on for medical care. Your primary doctor may be able to fulfill this role.

   While this may be adequate in many circumstances, we have found it beneficial to converse and rely on advice from other competent practitioners. They can give you a perspective that is "outside the box" of standard medical practice.

4. Gather your family and friends for support and find an appropriate support group. We have found that the support of family and friends is extremely beneficial.

   In addition, taking part in organized support groups helps everyone. Dr. Daniel Goleman has reported in his books that a significant amount of benefit can be gained from participation in support groups. Participating in such groups can improve longevity by as much as 40%.

5. Find out about the best possible lifestyle changes in diet, nutrition, supplements, and exercise that can improve your overall health. Lifestyle changes can be one of the most important factors for your recovery.

   Studies at the University of Massachusetts in the Mindfulness Based Stress Reduction program over the past 32 years have shown that opting for a vegetarian diet along with yoga and meditation practice can reduce symptoms and even help develop unexpected cures.

Dr. Dean Ornish has proven that the right kind of diet and exercise can reverse heart disease.
6. **Give back to your community when the time is right.** Your community supports your healing efforts and you will experience a lot of joy when you feel comfortable contributing to the benefit of others.
7. **Develop a daily mindfulness practice to cope with changes in physical, emotional, mental, and spiritual states with equanimity.** One of the best things you can do for yourself is to develop a daily meditation practice. It is possible to start with just nine minutes a day and build up to 30 or more minutes.

These principles are easy to adapt to just about any lifestyle. Most likely, you'll have to make some adjustments, however.

Taking on the attitude of becoming your own advocate for health care is an important way to begin. It is considered the entry point to the seven principles of **Mindfulness in Healing**, and probably really essential. Without this attitude, it can be difficult to embrace the other principles.

Each one is valuable in its own right and they all work together to enhance your life and create the best possible mindset for a complete recovery.

For example, exploring alternative and complementary care (i.e., integrative medicine, #2) does not require a healing professional that is familiar with both standard medical practices and integrative medicine (#3), but in my experience, having Michael Broffman at the Pine Street Clinic as my healing professional was a tremendous benefit.

I have found that my mindfulness practices have helped me integrate all seven of the principles of **Mindfulness in Healing**. In the pages that follow, you will discover how I used many mindfulness practices at various stages in my healing process.

One of the turning points occurred on the Vernal Equinox of 1997. I had a very powerful guided imagery session which served as the path for healing myself and inspiration to continue practicing. This imagery session was also the motivation for the title of the book and the cover image.

Other practices included sitting meditation, walking meditation, mindful movements, dance, creative writing and drawing, and meditation in bed when I couldn't do anything else. Being on retreat with Zen Master Thich Nhat Hanh came at a perfect time and provided me with a lot of love and support at a time when it was badly needed.

As I enter my seventeenth year of living with cancer, I find that meditation practices keep me on track with my healing experience and provide me with a refuge from fear, doubt, uncertainty, and worry. I feel that they are strong enough to help me embrace any situation I find myself in with regard to cancer and health issues.

Returning to my true home – my mindfulness of the present moment – relieves the stress of having to think about consequences, obstacles, and worst case scenarios. I stay on top of my feelings and this helps keep my family from feeling morose about my situation.

# INTRODUCTION

> *Lying still,*
> *Breathing in, breathing out,*
> *Healthy cells grow all by themselves.*
> *I am free of cancer!*

This Zen poem came to me during my guided imagery session on the day of the Vernal Equinox, 1997. It represents the theme of this document, which is also the title of the previous print version the book and the web site: *Healthy Cells Grow All By Themselves*. We have to be willing to allow our bodies to heal themselves by paying attention to our healing process, by paying attention to our breathing. We have to live moment by moment.

This book is devoted to cancer patients and other people facing difficult medical circumstances. It traces the symptoms and diagnosis of my bladder cancer from the onset of symptoms to Father's Day, 1996 and beyond. It is given in diary format so that other sufferers of the disease or any other disease can make use of my experience in whatever way is beneficial to them. Hopefully, my readers will be inspired to take an active role in their own recovery and be willing to participate in their own healing, rather than being at the mercy of the surgeon's knife. There is a considerable body of evidence that patients who have a positive mental attitude and engage in their own treatment have much better chance of long term survival.

Not everyone will want to do the amount of research I've done to find out about my disease, but if you do, this book should give you a good idea of where to start and what resources are available to help you participate in your on healing. I have incorporated a lot of alternative medicine and spiritual practices in my recovery, and I hope to inspire you to do the same.

There are a few bits of background information that you should know in order to understand my motivation for doing this in the way that it is being done.

First of all, I am a 74 year old male living in Marin County, California, one of the best places to live in the world, both from a pure aesthetic point of view, and because of its access to medical resources. The University of California at San Francisco Medical Center is just across the Golden Gate Bridge, and Stanford University Hospital is only fifty miles away. Furthermore, Marin General Hospital and its associated medical organizations are among the best in the country. So, right away, I feel that I am blessed to be living here.

Secondly, I am a person with a deep spiritual commitment. My orientation is Buddhist, and my interests lie in guided imagery ("*mind stories*"), cosmology, the enneagram, and conscious evolution. Being diagnosed with bladder cancer was a shock to my system of values, but the supportive community I live in combined with my Buddhist outlook has made this period of my life reasonably tolerable.

Thirdly, you should know that cancer runs rampant in my family. My younger sister, Judy died of Leukemia in 1968 at the age of 27. My father died of bladder cancer at the age of 86 and my mother died of another form of cancer at the age of 72. With all of this happening, you might think that I was "predisposed" to get the curse.

In addition, my son, Micah, now 45, survived a stage four Wilm's Tumor which he had in 1976. The key to his survival may have been the use of some of the alternative medical treatments, as the surgeon had given him up for dead. Even my surgeon said, "We weren't saving many stage fours in those days."

Micah's cancer had metastasized to his lungs and no one (perhaps except me) thought he would survive.

We were totally surprised when his doctors allowed us to use imagery and other alternative medical treatments with him. Micah and I worked together on *mind stories*, guided imagery sessions designed especially for children, from the first day he went into the hospital.

After he got out of the hospital, there were still rounds of chemotherapy and radiation he had to go through. There was also the wonderful Dr. Sheldon Ruderman who continued to do mind stories with Micah for many months.

My son's story was told in two episodes of "In Search of..." with Leonard Nimoy in 1976 and 1980. For more information about Micah's miraculous healing, please check out **Mind Stories Help Cure Cancer** on *Meditation Practices* (http://mountainsangha.org) website.

In the pages that follow, you will be able to trace my healing experience from the onset of disease to a complete recovery. Everything you read comes directly from my experience. Most of it is stream of consciousness writing as taught by Julia Cameron in *The Artist's Way*. I had been doing Morning Pages for many years prior and using the computer seemed like a good way to continue.

My hope is that you will benefit from seeing how one man **took charge of his own healing experience** and followed through on all types of treatments. I wish to inspire more people to participate in their health and healing by learning about their illness, following through with conventional medical treatments and considering alternatives to enhance their quality of life.

If only one person is helped by this book, my efforts will have been gratefully rewarded. Please help me spread the word of contributing to the well-being of all people.

Please note that since the writing was done in a stream of consciousness fashion, there are many places which would benefit from a skilled editor. I ask your forgiveness on this.

As you will read in the pages that follow, the technical term for the several surgeries I had is *transurethral resection of the bladder tumor* or TURBT in medical speak. It involves insertion of a device capable of removing visible cancer directly into the bladder through the urethra. While this may sound rather morbid, it beats abominable – oops I mean abdominal – surgery by leaps and bounds.

The radiation therapy was totally confined to my lower abdomen, specifically to my bladder. The chemotherapy was very rigorous and uncomfortable.

All three of these traditional medical practices were based on a bladder sparing protocol that I was lucky to find through a close friend who is a radiation oncologist.

The gold standard of medical practice for bladder cancer is to remove the bladder surgically, and replace it either with an artificial bladder or constructing a substitute using the patient's own bowel tissue. This did not appeal to me and I later learned that the complications of doing this procedure are horrendous.

# 1 - ONSET OF DISEASE

## 9/10/96: Red Stream

On September 10, 1996, I noticed that my urine was red. I immediately called my doctor and went over to have a urine specimen drawn. Yeah, there was blood in my urine all right, let's watch it for a few days and see what happens. The day after next, I had a clear stream, and a week later, there was no evidence of blood in my urine. Dr. Belknap thought that this could have been a blood vessel, or perhaps a kidney stone, but there was nothing to worry about.

## 12/22/96: More Red

By approximately December 22, 1996, I had two more innocuous episodes of blood in my urine, and made another appointment to see Dr. Belknap, but I could not see him until January 31 for a complete physical. As with the earlier episode, each of these cleared up in less than two days, so I was not worried.

## 1/21/96: Red Stream with Clots

On January 21, I once again had blood in my urine, accompanied by some clots. This one really scared me, but I knew I was seeing Dr. Belknap in ten days, so I did nothing, as the clots and bleeding stopped as quickly as it began.

## 1/26/96: Red River!

On Saturday night, January 25, I couldn't stop pissing blood. It was the most bewildering experience of my recent years. As I was unable to sleep, I started to surf the web for pages describing blood in the urine. The most interesting page I found was Hematuria from MedicineNet. It told me that hematuria could be gross or microscopic. Mine was of the super duper gross kind! Fortunately, I was able to sleep some after about two hours of surfing. Every time I got up though, I had to urinate and every time it was a red river. I was really worried by now. I woke up around 8:30 in the morning and called Dr. Belknap. I got his answering service and called the physician on duty, Dr. Jacoby. He set me up for an appointment at 10:45 on a Sunday morning! I then proceeded to phone Dr. Belknap at home, and he assured me that seeing Dr. Jacoby was the right thing to do.

After taking a urine sample, which, by the way, looked more like a blood sample, Dr. Jacoby examined my prostate gland and left the examination room to call the urologist on call at Marin General Hospital (the other *MGH!*) who happened to be Dr. Neuwirth. Dr. Jacoby strongly recommended that I head off to the hospital so that Dr. Neuwirth could run some tests to see what was causing all this blood.

We arrived at the emergency room of MGH at around 11:30, armed with a bag containing the urine sample, in perfect time to meet Dr. Neuwirth. Can you imagine not having to wait four hours in the waiting room! He walked away with the bag and returned in less the 10 seconds. "I want to admit you and do some tests," he said.

After that, in short fashion, I found myself in a typical hospital gown, lying in bed with an IV started in my left wrist. In less than an hour I had X-rays, a CT scan, and an intravenous pyelogram, or IVP, which is an x-ray evaluation of the urinary tract. All of these tests were expected due to the excellent coverage of the hematuria web page.

The results were not favorable. From the CT scan, it was obvious that I had some kind of tumor at the base of the bladder and therefore a cystoscopy was necessary. This was to be scheduled as soon as possible, but actually would never take place on Super bowl Sunday! What medical team would be willing to give up their Sunday evening, anyway?

So there I was, back in my bed, just in time to watch the Super bowl. By then, the phone was ringing off of the hook, and my friend, Dr. Rossman came to visit me to look into my condition. He is an outstanding physician in his own right and specializes in interactive guided imagery, and acupuncture. He brought with him a new guided imagery tape for pre-operative patients in which he collaborated with Stephen Halprin. I also had a few other visitors, including my sister and her husband, my son, and another good friend. I think the gentleman I was sharing the room with was getting fed up with all of the phone calls. I knew I had a tremendous support group behind me. This, by the way, is one of the important factors in helping yourself to a speedy recovery - having a support group of people who love you unconditionally.

After everyone left, I settled down and listened to Dr. Rossman's tape. This helped me to relax and visualize some long range goals, such as playing tennis four days a week once again. With meditation and visualization techniques, I was able to sleep most of the night, barring interruptions from nurses who wanted to suck more of my blood.

One interesting thing that happened that night was that one of the nurses wanted me to sign my operation consent from. After reading it over, I decided that I needed to speak with an anesthesiologist first, in order to determine whether I should go with a general anesthetic or an epidural. The nurse said that he would get one up to my room, but one never came. The next nurse on duty also tried to get me to sign, but I still refused. It took them until 3:00 P. M. the next day for one to come, and I missed an opportunity for a 9:00 A. M. surgery.

## 1/27/97: TURBT

My refusal to sign the operation afforded me another whole day of waiting. In the morning, I had visits from Dr. Belknap and Dr. Neuwirth, both of which were very helpful in pointing out the pros and cons of the alternative anesthetic methods, but I still hadn't made up my mind. I wanted to speak with an expert.

Dr. Neuwirth tried to prepare me for the best case scenario, which would involve complete resection of the bladder tumor followed by quarterly inspections with a cystoscopy and possibly coupled with chemotherapy agents inserted directly in the bladder. I found this discussion rather informative, but would have preferred a more accurate reading of my tumor.

Since my daughter was ill, my wife couldn't be with me the whole time, so I spent the day receiving phone calls and visitors, and listening to classical music, and Dr. Rossman's tape. Since I couldn't eat or drink, my thoughts continually turned to food, especially when my roommate ate his meals. In between time, I continued my meditation and visualization practices, which kept me from getting to anxious about the ensuing operation.

At around 3:00 P. M., my wife returned to the hospital, just in time for the meeting with the anesthesiologist. His name was Christophe Dannello and he was very nice. He carefully explained the various options, and with his guidance, I decided to go with the epidural.

Around 6:30 P.M., they came to wheel me off to surgery. I grabbed Dr. Rossman's tape and headed off to the operating room. I was given a sedative intravenously and placed on the table. A moment later, a small needle was applied to my lower back and I was turned over and placed into position. The oxygen feeder was placed in my nose and my legs were positioned in place for the surgery.

Then... I was gone! I woke up in the recovery room and spent what seemed like only fifteen minutes there. I was taken back to my room and my wife was with me for the next half-hour or so. Then she had to get home to the children, so there I was, lying flat on my back with a catheter in me. I started to feel pain from the epidural and was given "candy" - vicodin. This controlled the pain.

I proceeded to do my "mind story" and had a fairly good night sleep until I was rudely awakened for vital signs around midnight. Luckily, the rest of the night was uneventful, even though I was leaking blood through my catheter.

## 1/28/97: Going Home!

I was awakened the next morning at around 6:00 A. M. by ... guess who? A nurse of course who wanted my vital signs and other data. The catheter was supposed to be removed by 7:00 A. M., but the nurses decided to wait until Dr. Neuwirth showed up and voiced his opinion.

I was visited in rapid succession by Dr. Belknap and Dr. Neuwirth. The latter found the nurses' objection to removing the catheter rather lame and ten minutes later it was gone. I asked him, "On a scale of one to ten, how do you rate the surgery?" His reply, as he got up to leave, was, "Ten, of course! I always do ten!"

There wasn't much else he could tell me until the biopsy was completed and the pathology report issued. Apparently, he was able to remove all of the tumor that was visible above the muscle layer of the bladder and he also removed additional samples around the tumor and at remote sites.

A few hours later, I was on my way home! What a shock! Four days earlier I was playing tennis. Now I was laid up for approximately three to four weeks, and I was still pissing blood. What else lay in store for me?

Fortunately, there were a large number of well-wishers calling, sending cards, and stopping by. When I arrived home, there was a gorgeous bouquet waiting for me on the porch. It turned out to be from the RND group at NGC! I was really touched by their efforts and concern.

That night, I suffered tremendously from the pain of the epidural.

However, one call to Christophe gave me the information I needed to relieve the pain. He suggested three Motrin along with the vicodin.

**1/29/97: Radical Is As Radical Does!**

Around noon on this day, I received a phone call from Dr. Neuwirth. He wanted to see me in his office at 5:00 P. M. that afternoon. He also told me that I had a bladder cancer and that he needed to explain to me all of my options.

Instead of panicking, I immediately started a search on the World Wide Web for "bladder cancer." I found many references and lots of good sites. I printed off several of them to take with me to Dr. Neuwirth's office. These included *Bladder Cancer*, *Understanding Bladder Cancer*, MedicineNet's *Bladder Cancer*, and About Bard BTA Test. Of these, the first turned out to be the most useful because of the way it talks about treatment by stage of bladder cancer.

We brought R. D., the father of a childhood friend of my wife, and Dr. Rossman to the meeting with Dr. Neuwirth to help us remember the conversation and all that we said. It is always a good idea to take people you trust so that they can bear witness to your conversation and possibly hear things that you can't because of your emotional involvement with the case.

Dr. Neuwirth started to explain the "stage" and "grade" of the tumor based on a preliminary verbal report from the pathologist. Once he said "T2," I dropped the Bladder Cancer paper pointing to the section on T2-4 tumors. His jaw practically fell to his desk! He said, "I wouldn't put it that bluntly, but that's basically what we have here!" He also mentioned that I had some carcinoma-in-situ and a bit of dysplasia, which are abnormal cells. Later, we found out that I also had some atypia cells from Dr. Torigoe (see below).

He proceeded to explain the ins and outs of the medical alternatives for treatment of stage two bladder cancer. The choices were basically

1. Cystectomy - partial or radical
2. Radiation
3. Chemotherapy

Dr. Neuwirth, being a surgeon, naturally recommended radical cystectomy. We asked him all of the questions in Appendix 1. [**NOTE:** The questions for this appendix can be found on the ***Mindfulness In Healing*** website at http://mindfulnessinhealing.org/appendix-1.]

My son was born on January 29, 1969. Today he was 28 years old. It's funny how life is. I had to give him the bad news on his birthday. On March 7, 9, 14, and 16 he was scheduled to have a leading role in La Boheme, as Marcello. I wanted to see him perform and didn't want any disabling therapy to begin before I had a chance to see him.

That night, we spoke with Dr. Sara Huang, a radiation oncologist at St. Mary's Hospital in San Francisco. She has long been a friend of the family and was devastated by the news. She mentioned that the "Gold Standard" of treatment for bladder cancer was radical cystectomy. However, she had some hopeful information about the possibility of chemotherapy used in conjunction with radiation therapy and recommend that we consult Dr. Wayne Torigoe at Marin General.

## 2 - TREATMENT OPTIONS

### 1/30/97: Radiological Consult

The next day we met with Dr. Torigoe. This time we took J and L with us. They have been friends for the whole time my wife and I have been together, and they have and extremely rational outlook on life.
Naturally, we would have liked to take Dr. Rossman too, but he has his practice and we didn't want to bother him.

We had a very long discussion with Dr. Torigoe. His patience and understanding were remarkable. He, too, thought that the "Gold Standard" for treatment of bladder cancer is radical cystectomy. But, as he put it, "Radiation and chemotherapy are a viable alternative, especially if the radical cystectomy is too morbid for some people."

When I explained what transpired in our conversation with Dr. Torigoe to Dr. Rossman, he recommended that I contact Dr. Dave Gullion, who he was planning to see the next day at Commonweal. Dr. Gullion is a medical oncologist in the same building as Dr. Torigoe and he is also associated with Marin General Hospital.

### 1/31/97: Yellow Stream!!

On the morning of January 31, 1997, I finally had what looked like a normal yellow stream! I was so excited that it made my day. Another great thing that happened that morning is that M. C. gave me a check for four therapeutic massages with Elyse, whom we've been seeing for over a year.

Around 11:00, R. M. called me to have lunch with J. M. J. was diagnosed with prostate cancer several years ago, but appears to be in remission now, with only natural medicine regimes. His PSA test is normal now, but he has had to work hard and be careful with his diet. Luckily, J. M. has the resources to fly all over the country to find the best alternative medical treatments.

J.'s original reaction to my situation was to recommend radical cystectomy. However, having the night before to look through his library of books on cancer, he had changed his mind by the time he picked me up to go to lunch. We discussed all the alternative healers that J. had visited, but much of his treatment didn't apply to me, since prostate cancer is much slower growing. Overall, it was wonderful to have the support of someone who has had to deal with the same emotional issues when confronted with having cancer.

Later that afternoon, three members of my evolutionary circle visited me and they proceeded to perform a healing circle for my benefit. It was shortly after they left that I named this we site, "Yellow Stream!"

After they left, I had time to look at the papers that were sent over by Dr. Huang. One of these papers was delivered on my 55th birthday in 1995 and bore the name of William U. Shipley. I spent much of the rest of the afternoon tracking down other works by Shipley and his associates and ultimately finding the phone number of his son. I phoned Shipley's son and pleaded my case to him. He agreed to notify his father and possibly have him call me.

Later that day, I phone Dr. Neuwirth to see if he knew of Dr. Shipley. He said, "Shipley - Oh yes, the bladder saving guru!" I was excited that this man was known even to a local Urologist! Just before we got off the phone, I asked Dr. Neuwirth if he had a copy of the completed pathology report that he could fax to me. He said that he did and he would.

## 2/1/97: Shipley: The Bladder Saving Guru

Early Saturday morning, I received a phone call from Dr. Shipley, which we almost missed!!! However, since I already had his office number, I called back immediately, and the nurse relayed the message to him, for he called back a few minutes later.

The conversation revolved around likely candidates for the Shipley approach, which combines chemotherapy and radiation therapy in an effort to save the bladder. He explained how his protocol involved four weeks of chemotherapy combined with radiation, followed by four weeks off. At the end of the second four week period, a cystoscopy is performed to look for the presence of tumors. If tumors are found, the radical cystectomy is recommended. If none are found, another four weeks of chemotherapy and radiation are applied and the bladder is followed up with cystoscopy examinations every three to four months. Subsequent local superficial growths are handled with intravesical chemotherapy using BCG or mitomycin, in which the chemotherapeutic agents are instilled directly in the bladder.

Dr. Shipley discussed how they like to work with patients who have had all the tumor removed with TURBT, as his success rate increases when this is the case. As I wasn't sure if Dr. Neuwirth had resected all of the tumor, my hopes were a bit dimmed. He even mentioned that they sometimes use cystoscopy and transurethral resection two or three times to make sure they got all of the tumor.

This conversation gave me some hope. He even stated that I could come to Boston for a consultation with himself, along with Dr. Kaufman and Dr. Heney. Shipley referred to Marin General Hospital as, "The other 'MGH'!" and mentioned the names of Dr. Francine Halberg and Dr. Patrick Bennett. Dr. Bennett had trained with Dr. Shipley and his team of oncologists and urologists and Shipley regards him as his protégé. So the next obvious thing was to speak with Dr. Bennett.

I had originally phoned Dr. Bennett when he was on call just after my surgery to ask him what to do about my back pain. He was quite helpful then, and during the conversation I had with him after speaking with Shipley he was also very nice and understanding. He told me what I already knew about the Shipley approach in that it worked best with all of the cancer resected, but that he would have to discuss my case with Dr. Neuwirth.

This was the day of many visitors and phone calls from well-wishers. For example, J. D. brought us dinner from Kitty's place and brought me a copy of Andy Weil's book, *Spontaneous Healing*, which I have been reading ever since. Late in the evening, Dr. Rossman phoned me to tell me that he had spoken with Dr. Gullion, Dr. Keith Block (from Evanston, IL), and John Boik, author of an excellent book on cancer research and alternatives.

## 2/2/97: Should I Ship off to Shipley?

The next morning, I had a very interesting conversation with Dr. Huang about Shipley. She was quite impressed that I not only tracked Shipley down, but that I actually spoke with him. I had faxed a copy of the pathology report the day before. She had always been a proponent of the Shipley method in my case, but now, armed with the pathology report, she was even more confident. She even recommended that I make the trip to Boston to consult with Shipley and his team.

Later that morning, Dr. Rossman came by with John Boik's book. We spoke a bit about the options, be Dr. Rossman has a habit of throwing decisions back on people, with expressions such as, "What do you think?"

That day was filled with many visitors and phone calls. One phone call that I made was to P. F. We had been to her birthday party on the night the "Red River" started to flow, and I know that P. was involved with a Russian healer. During the conversation, she gave me Nicholi's phone number and I set up and appointment with him for the next Tuesday. More about this man later.

## 2/3/97: Oncological Consult

Finally, one of my girls was recovered from the horrible virus that has struck our community, but we still had the other one at home. Having the girls around makes strategic conversations a little difficult.
However, we were scheduled into Dr. Gullion this morning and I got T. W. from my conscious evolution group to stay with J. J. and L. once again consented to be present at the consultation with us.

We sat down with Dr. Gullion and he was wearing a pin shaped like a heart over his pocket. He was tall and had a very welcoming smile. However, due to the seriousness of my illness, he was a bit serious himself. He sent the others out of the room for a few minutes while he examined me.

When the others returned to the room, he asked me what was wrong (as if he didn't know) and I explained that I had a stage four bladder cancer that was highly active along with carcinoma in situ and some dysplasia and atypia cells. He was impressed with my understanding, and proceeded to write out my diagnosis and treatment alternatives "Patient Communication Sheet."

You have: Papillary transitional cell carcinoma, Grade IV/IV T2 (T3a), No, Mo

Treatment:
1. Radical Cystectomy - standard therapy
2. Neoadjuvant therapy - Bladder sparing
3. Chemotherapy - MCV x 2 cycles followed by radiation: 4000 rads with cisplatin (2 cycles). Then re-evaluate with cystoscopy and biopsy. If (-) - radiation - close follow-up. If (+) - surgery.

While this was slightly different than the Shipley protocol as I understood it, I could see that he had done his homework after speaking with Dr. Rossman.

We continued to ask questions (see Appendix 2 [**NOTE**: The questions for this appendix can be found on the ***Mindfulness In***

*Healing* website at http://mindfulnessinhealing.org/appendix-2.]), and left with the feeling that radical cystectomy was the way to go. We discussed both options with J. and L. over lunch. During that time, I decided to go to their house with them in order to use their Jacuzzi bathtub. As we passed the tennis courts, I was filled with grief, as I surely would rather be playing tennis. That night I was starting to come down with a cold, which my wife treated homeopathically.

**2/4/97: No Magic Bullets**

The next morning, we shipped J. off with M. L. T. and headed for Dr. Roger Morrison, a world renowned homeopath. We explained the situation to Roger, and he was all for the bladder saving approach, especially because it provided an option to save the bladder, as well as a fallback position of bladder removal. However, we didn't learn very much new from Roger, and this was rather disappointing. We were looking for a magic bullet, but none was to be found.

In the afternoon, I saw the Russian healer, Nicholi Levaschov, in San Francisco. I loved the man at first sight, as I could see his healing qualities and felt good in his presence. However, I found it very difficult to understand his English, and therefore have not followed up with any further treatment, as yet. What he did was quite remarkable, though. He seemed to be able to stand over my body and evoke healing energy. He moved his hands in circles around the area of my bladder, and I felt the energy quite clearly. I sensed that he was working with colors and when I felt the color, yellow, I made a comment. He confirmed my sensitivity and continued the treatment. All in all, I was there for about thirty minutes and enjoyed the experience quite well.

My next appointment was with Suzanne Schmidt's healer, Yokey Kim, at his studio, Kim's Yoga Body Design in Japan Town in San Francisco. Kim is a Korean shiatsu and acupressure healer of top quality. I felt a lot of tension release from my shoulders and legs during the treatment, which lasted about one hour. The cost of the session was only forty dollars!

Although Roger, Nicholi, and Kim are all incredible natural healers, there were no magic bullets to be had! I was left to my own devices, such as "mind stories" and other spiritual practices.

**2/5/97: Pissing Contest**

M. L. T. picked up J. so that we could meet with Dr. Peter Carroll, the Oncological Urologist that everyone said was the best in the Bay Area. L. C. met us at the U. C. Medical Center in his office. After a brief case history and yet another prostate exam, Dr. Carroll once again explained the standard of treatment for bladder cancer: radical cystectomy. We were encouraged by his some two hundred bladder removals and eighty urinary diversion operations. We felt that this was the man to do any cutting, if any was to be done. We asked him all the questions in Appendix 2 [**NOTE**: The questions for this appendix can be found on the **Mindfulness In Healing** website at http://mindfulnessinhealing.org/appendix-2.]. We left there feeling confident that Dr. Carroll could handle any surgery that I might need.

Later that afternoon, I saw my therapist, Suzanne Schmidt for the first time since November. She was going through some radical changes in healing herself, which included almost daily visits to Yokey Kim. We started a new therapy involving self-massage of the chakras (seven energy points within the body described by Indian yogis) and the mental and emotional pain associated with them. We were quite in synch during the whole session, which lasted over two hours. We seemed to be healing each other, but I still did not get a clear idea of how to treat my bladder cancer. I left her house feeling very good!

Suzanne had recommended that I try to see Kim every day, if possible, so when I got home I called him. He said that I could come in at 6:00 P. M., which I did. The second treatment was better than the first, in that I was more relaxed and knew what to expect.

## 2/6/97: The Big Surprise!

The next morning, my wife and I had another helpful conversation with Sara Huang. Once again, she was emphasizing the possibility of saving my bladder, but we were predisposed to think about surgery.

Then came our consultation with Dr. Gullion who had the tumor board results from early in the morning. To our shock, amazement and surprise, the tumor board came to the decision that I could take my choice between radical cystectomy and the Shipley treatment! They felt that the entire visible tumor **had** been removed by Dr. Neuwirth and my chances were the same with either treatment. We were stunned! We had no idea that this would be the result of the tumor board! Now what was I going to do? See appendix 3 for the questions we asked Dr.

Gullion. [**NOTE:** The questions for this appendix can be found on the ***Mindfulness In Healing*** website at http://mindfulnessinhealing.org/appendix-3.]

One thing was clear: I didn't want abominable surgery! After speaking with Dr. Belknap about the results of the tumor board, I received a call from J. W., a close friend of mine from my enneagram centers group. She had gone through surgery and chemotherapy for ovarian cancer and was finally beginning to feel more like herself. I asked her what she thought of my two options, and she said that abdominal surgery was horrible. She would vote for the chemo and radiation. I liked her reasoning and knew that she was speaking personal experience.

Joan also gave me advice in the following areas. She suggested that I check with my insurance company to see if I was covered for a social worker to come in the house and help out when I was going through the worse part of chemotherapy. She also said the cisplatin was very hard on the kidneys and that I should allow for eight hours of rehydration. She prepared me for short-term memory loss during chemotherapy, and wanted to make sure that I had a cocktail of drugs. The typical Shipley treatment is to apply cisplatin with methyltrexate and vinblastine together, so I may not have to worry about this. However, she was careful to emphasize that I should carefully check what is being fed into me because there have been many cases of chemotherapy overdoses! She cautioned me to stay away from anti-nausea drugs and use sea-bands instead. She recommended getting a hold of the National Cancer Institute (1-800-4-CANCER) for specific information about the drugs I'll be taking and how to best deal with the side effects. She recommended taking caraloe and aloe vera combination with vitamin E and suggested that I read, "*The Chemotherapy Survival Guide.*"

By the time I finished my conversation with Joan, I was on my way to my decision not to have radical cystectomy.

### 2/7/97: I Don't Want Abominable Surgery!

Friday morning, I had to have a sonogram for my gall stone. Aside from the long wait, it went fairly smoothly. When I finished, my friend, T. R. was waiting for me. We had breakfast together and talked about my options.

After T. left for work, I joined a cancer support group at Marin General led by Leslie Davenport. She had worked with my wife the previous year doing guided imagery for her hip problem that was caused by an automobile accident in 1992. I was the only man, but this didn't stop me from trying to find out what was the best course of action. One of the women said that she had no side effects from the chemotherapy whatever!

In the early afternoon, I had another session with Yokey Kim. Once again, I had a wonderful treatment.

Then came the long-awaited appointment with Michael Broffman, a Chinese herbalist and acupuncturist, who runs the Pine Street Clinic. He has a fabulous reputation for knowing a lot about cancer, and my wife and I were blown away by his knowledge of bladder cancer. We talked at great length about alternatives to radical cystectomy. One surprising note was something that no other physician mentioned. Michael said that after seven or more years, they may have to go in for another operation for the urinary diversion. After this statement, decision was really moving rapidly towards the Shipley approach! Michael proceeded to tell us that there is a lot of bladder cancer in China and that a combination of traditional Chinese medicine and chemotherapy, with or without radiation, is the primary means of dealing with the disease.

By the time we left Michael's office, we felt comfortable that the Shipley method combined with the protocol Michael was going to send us would offer me a better chance than just the Shipley method alone.

### 2/8/97: What Kind of Day was This?

Saturday morning, I received a phone call from R. M. that Suzanne was ill and that R. and I were to lead the workshop that was scheduled for 11:00. This was really weird! We had to improvise most of the morning, but somehow, we managed. Several people, including myself, explained how Suzanne's "new therapy" worked and how they felt about it.

After the strange workshop, I had my first walk outdoors since the surgery. Boy! Did it make me exhausted. When we got home, I really had to listen to my body and I took a long nap.

### 2/9/97: A Vietnamese Buddhist Physician Acupuncturist

Elyse came to my house to give me one of her wonderful massages that

M. C. paid for. It was relaxing and very enjoyable.

In the middle of the afternoon, I went to see a Vietnamese Buddhist acupuncturist, Van Vu (H 25), who spends his Sundays in Mill Valley. He was very perceptive and stated that while I had good chi, I had too much hate inside, and suffered from bad sleep. He was right on!

That night, we all had dinner with J. and L. C. - the ones who had been so helpful at the consultations with the physicians - and no mention was made about treatment options. We just had a good time and over ate her wonderful sesame chicken recipe!

## 3 - MAKING THE DECISION
### 2/10/97: Moving Toward Health

Up until now, I have been reporting on external events and meetings with physicians. It has certainly been a whirlwind of activity for the last two weeks, but I haven't mentioned too much of what is going on inside. Believe me, a lot is taking place and has transpired. I have continued to do "mind stories" daily, sometimes three or more times a day, especially when I feel tired. While the method I use to invoke the relaxed state of mind that I need to do my meditation is described elsewhere, the content of my meditation is made up of at least three kinds of processes.

The first process I use is based on Buddhist meditation. Having been trained in both Zen and Vipassana, I use a hybrid method that incorporates the best of both for my purposes. The method involves following the breath in the belly, which is a common practice in both Zen and Vipassana, with a healing twist. What I used to do prior to my diagnosis was "breathing in ... breathing out" - following the physical movement of my abdomen. The modification I make, based on the teachings of Thich Nhat Hanh, along with bringing my attention a little lower to my bladder, I generally repeat, "Breathing in, I know that I am healing myself, ... breathing out, the cancer is gone!" Much of the time, when the breath is fairly short, for example, I use the trigger words, "healing" for the in breath and "gone" for the out breath, knowing that I am referring to the elimination of the cancer cells.

The second method is to visualize the insides of my bladder, and visualize that I am scraping off the cancer cells into the bladder, to be easily eliminated through normal bladder function. This is a quite effective technique, as sometimes I really feel the cells dying and being eliminated. This process takes a good deal of concentration to be effective, but many years of visualization practice have helped in this area.

The third method is to visualize events in my future with a positive regard. For example, I see myself playing tennis in Sausalito, Edgewood Park and Boyle Park, with my different tennis buddies. Or, I might see myself lying on China Beach in Point Lobos State Reserve, and listening to the waves crash against the shore. I can smell the sea air and virtually taste the salt water. I feel the texture of the sand on my feet, legs, buttocks, hands, and arms. Or, I might visualize R.'s graduation coming up in June or a trip to Hawaii, or whatever my mind brings up. I'm not focusing on my disease at all, as these events take me beyond recovery.

Why, you may wonder, am I bringing all of this up today? Well, after spending the day requesting the Shipley protocol and ordering all of the ingredients in Michael Broffman's protocol, I attended a support group led by Anna Halprin. Anna is a dancer in her late seventies that diagnosed and treated her own cancer with movement and art. Twenty-one years ago, I studied with Gabrielle Roth, one of Anna's protégés, so I was familiar with her work. I also attended a retrospective performance by Anna and her students about a year ago. I was very excited to attend her group this evening because I hadn't been allowed to play tennis since before the "red stream."

Anna's group consisted of mostly women who had already recovered from cancer. There were several ladies who were in the throes of treatment, but they were in the minority. Anna began by allowing my friend J. M. (the same friend who took me to lunch after "yellow stream") to tell his story of three and one half years of prostate cancer which is no in total remission. Everyone was encouraged by his story.

She proceeded to direct us to get grounded in our chairs and begin breathing in and out. Naturally, my Buddhist practice came to mind and I was in a rhythm of "healing... gone." We then started moving in time with our breath, expanding way out with our arms open wide on the in breath and contracting inward on the out breath. This theme was developed to standing, bending, and movement around the room to Native American music of some kind. We eventually had some group interaction through the movement and all along Anna kept us focused on our breath. She would have us focus on being grounded, relaxed, aware, centered energy (grace).

After the period of movement, we were to draw a picture inspired by the movement. This was a difficult task for me, for I have never enjoyed drawing too much. With her inspiration and support, I drew the "yellow stream."

## 2/11/97: Decision Day

In the morning, I spoke with Dr. Gullion over the phone and told him that I wanted to follow the Shipley treatment precisely. He said it would be no problem. I also spoke with him about Michael Broffman's protocol. While he cautioned me about taking antioxidants during the first several days of chemotherapy, he was willing to cooperate. I explained to him that Michael had broken the protocol down into three parts, as described above, and he seemed to feel better about that.

In the afternoon, I had a guided imagery session with Dr. Martin Rossman. The session followed a discussion about my treatment options and the one I selected. Marty had been following my choices since day one, so he was familiar with what I was going through. He thought that I made the right decision, and that I had a lot of additional things going for me.

The guided imagery session was extremely relaxing. It encouraged me to experience reality based anchoring in my body, which I did in a big way. I contacted my "inner advisor" and got in touch with a sense of deep spirituality. From the vantage point of a grove of trees in Point Lobos State Reserve, I was able to feel my connection with the earth and really felt good. My illness seemed thousands of miles away, as I was able to ground myself in what I was experiencing in the moment. I felt that for me, a strong sense of integrity is directly connected with listening to my body and acting accordingly.

As deep as the session with Marty had taken me, I became confused after taking a long walk and picking up the kids from school. After speaking with my wife about the events of the day, I was experiencing a lot of pressure to begin the therapy as soon as possible - like February 17, when I had it in my mind to begin February 24. I decided to take the evening off and watch public television which portrayed the magnificent engineering accomplishments at Stonehenge and of the Incas.

## 2/12/97: Back to Work

This morning I spoke with Francine Halberg, a colleague of Dr. Wayne Torigoe. She knew who I was because she had already spoken with Dr. Gullion and Dr. Shipley! She wants to see me to discuss the difficulties and side effects of Dr. Shipley's regime.

On the way to NGC, I listened to a tape of a lecture by Dr. Allen Hoffman in which he spoke about his work with a concentrated form Aloe Vera and the use of cesium chloride in the treatment of AIDS and cancer. The lecture was very understandable, and I want to see if he is simply selling, "snake oil!" Later that evening, I spoke with P. R. and Dr. Huang about is, but was unable to get any further information.

## 2/13/97: More Resection?

I called Dr. Hoffman this morning and spoke with him about the treatment of bladder cancer with cesium chloride and/or aloe vera concentrate, and he basically said that these were not to replace chemotherapy and radiation. This was confirmed by a later conversation with Michael Broffman, who knew of Dr. Hoffman, and told us that Dr. Hoffman's protocol was something to consider at the end of the Shipley treatments.

Then we received a call from Dr. Neuwirth. He said that Dr. Gullion had called him about the Shipley method, which requires an additional transurethral resection of the bladder tumor (TURBT), which he wanted to schedule for next week. We spoke to Michael Broffman about this and he recommended that we talk to Dr. Carroll. After further discussions with Dr. Huang, Dr. Gullion, we finally received a call back from Dr. Carroll. He said that he was out of time next week and the week after, so he wouldn't be able to do anything until the week of February 24. He suggested that I go with Dr. Neuwirth, whom he said was a competent surgeon and could do this job effectively.

The last time I had a TURBT, there was no plan to do anything other than a radical cystectomy. Now Dr. Neuwirth would go in with the idea of doing bladder saving therapy. This could account for Dr. Neuwirth's apparent reticence to do the second round of resection.

## 2/14/97: Happy Anniversary!

Today, Mala and I celebrated our sixteenth anniversary. We did this by heading up to the famous "wine county" in Napa County, California. We are so fortunate to live only 45 minutes from this most beautiful part of the country. Mala had made reservations at the Silverado Inn, which we were lucky to get at the last minute. With lunch at Don Giovanni's and dinner at Tra Vigne, we had two wonderful meals at our favorite places.

Before heading north, however, we met with Dr. Francine Halberg at the Marin Oncology Center attached to Marin General Hospital. Through Sara Huang's guidance and support, we decided to use Dr.

Halberg for the radiation therapy, which is scheduled to begin on February 25, along with the chemotherapy. The consultation with Dr. Halberg went very well as far as it could go, but she couldn't tell me that this was going to be an easy protocol (RTOG 95-06). She mentioned that Shipley had great success with this protocol and that it was evaluated thoroughly in France and found to be very successful. She explained that I would have to be seen again on Tuesday, February 18 to do a test run to map out the area to be irradiated, which was part of the RTOG 95-06 protocol.

Before we left for the "wine country," we stopped in the Circle Library at the Marin Oncology Center and checked out a few tapes, including one by Dr. Carl Simonton, whose work was just beginning to be noticed when my son had cancer twenty-one years ago. Another tape was by Dr. Rachel Naomi

### 2/15/97: No Doctors!

Today was one of the first days without appointments. Although I felt rested when we left the Inn, I felt rather down and low on energy all day. We walked around St. Helena and ate lunch at Don Giovanni's again. When I got home, I listened to a Simonton tape, and got totally recharged!

### 2/16/97: Another Day of Massage and Acupuncture!

I woke up early this morning with the idea to improve the web site by adding the practice pages. I got fairly far with the basic relaxation technique when it became time for my massage with Elyse. She is so wonderful! How lucky I am to listen to the best music and have a wonderful massage!

Just before my massage, my back started hurting, and by the time I got to Dr. Vu, it was hurting pretty badly. His treatment helped a lot, but because of the nature of my cancer treatment plans, I don't know when I'll be able to see him again.

I spent the evening reviewing the literature from T-Up, visiting with friends, reading Dr. Siegel's book and listening to meditation tapes.

### 2/17/97: More Moving Towards Health

This morning, I had a Feldenkrais lesson with G. T., a friend of my through D. B. It was preliminary lesson breathing and was followed by a short Functional Integration session. Both of these experiences were comforting and relaxing.

After taking R. to her friend's house, I decided to try playing tennis and managed to play two sets without too much strain. It was wonderful to be out on the court again. One hardly realizes the value of activities one loves until it becomes inaccessible!

That night, I returned to Anna Halprin's group at Marin General Hospital. It was another healing experience. The theme of the evening was water, and I immediately got an image of a waterfall I had seen in a photograph or movie. The water was flowing over the edge of a cliff in such a way that there was a substantial overhang, and one could walk through the waterfall and be protected from the water underneath the overhang. I drew a picture of this scene and wrote the following:

*Here we have stupid Ninad -*
*He thinks that because he is empty of self that he is also empty of suffering and that suffering is empty of self!*
*Wait until next week!!*
*He'd rather be surfing (the web) rather than suffering.*
*He should learn to step on the rocks, stupid!*

A little explanation is called for here. In the drawing; (which I shall try to scan someday), there is a picture of three stones that one would step on to walk into the waterfall. While I was drawing the rocks, I was reminded of the joke about Jesus, Buddha and Moses. They were walking across the Jordan River one day and Moses kept sinking deeper and deeper into the water, but Buddha and Jesus had no problem staying on the surface. When Jesus saw Moses sinking, he yelled back to him, "Step on the rocks, stupid!" The reference to my personal life was simple: I should "step on the rocks" of those who have gone before me with the treatment of bladder cancer. However, this is not my nature. I want to know what's happening and have some control of my life.

The name, Ninad, was given to me by Bhagwan Shree Rajneesh in 1975 - before he was famous. He explained to me that "Ninad" means the *sound of the waterfall!*

## 2/18/97: Treatment Delayed!

Mala and I went to visit Dr. Halberg again today for a simulation run through of the radiation therapy that was supposed to have begun on

February 25. However, Dr. Halberg had spoken with Dr. Shipley and was told that the chemotherapy and radiation treatments shouldn't begin until three weeks after the TURBT. So, I'm off the hook for three more weeks! I wasn't terribly surprised, because the protocol, itself says that registration begins three to four weeks post TURBT.

Dr. Halberg also reported that I had a urinary tract infection, and I was put on Cipro for the next two weeks.

Next, we went to Marin General Hospital to register for the TUR tomorrow. While this was time consuming, it was not particularly unpleasant.

I spent most of the rest of the day preparing my legal documents, including a Durable Power of Attorney for Health Care, which is a good document to have for your own protection.

## 4 - TREATMENT PREPARATIONS

### 2/19/97: Another TURBT

I went into the hospital early this morning to have another TURBT procedure done by Dr. Neuwirth. I was taken into the operating room about 75 minutes early, along with Dr. Rossman's pre surgery tape! This time, I was not given the opportunity to have an epidural. Instead, I had a general anesthetic. Luckily, I did not experience any side effects from the anesthetic.

My recovery was a little uncomfortable this time, probably because of the catheter, but maybe from the anesthetic. I was rolled up into my room about noon time and immediately started drinking. I wanted to flush out the disease from my bladder as soon as possible. In between visitors, I spent the afternoon comfortably doing "mind stories", listening to tapes by Dr. Keith Block and Dr. Carl Simonton, and reading *Love, Medicine and Miracles*. Later that evening, E. M. and D. F., two of my favorite tennis partners, came by. It was so nice to speak with them about how I use tennis as a spiritual practice and introduces them to visualization and guided imagery.

My wife is very clever! She talked Dr. Neuwirth into letting me spend the night in the hospital, which is not normally done after a TURBT. I was grateful for the overnight stay because I don't have to deal with a catheter until Tuesday.

### 2/20/97: Home Again!

The morning in the hospital was fairly uneventful. I continued to read and listen to tapes until Dr. Neuwirth showed up. When he did, he explained that he took more tissue out of the bladder wall and left me with a very thin membrane. To help the healing, he wanted me to keep the catheter in until Tuesday. However, he didn't seem to find any more gross cancer during the TURBT. Although the catheter is rather uncomfortable, I was very excited that there was no more visible tumor in my bladder! He was even telling me to "fatten up" for the chemotherapy that was going to happen in three weeks. I got the impression that he was satisfied with my decision to go with the Shipley method.

I spent the afternoon completing the "mind story" on the practice pages and submitting my URL to the various search engines. Somehow, time seems to flow so much faster now. My guess is that once you are confronted with a life-threatening illness, you value each minute a lot more. For example, when I played tennis on Monday, I thought it was very precious time, as I don't know when the next time I'll be able to play. Another example: M.'s cooking today seemed to be extra special.

### 2/21/97: A Day at Home

I had a fairly restful night considering that I had to take care of my own catheter! It was interesting to not to have to get up to pee! The catheter, however, kept me rather confined. It's amazing how rapidly it fills up!

I spent the day talking with visitors, speaking on the phone, and emptying my bag!

### 2/22/97: Practice What You Preach!

Today was an interesting day! I was feeling kind of down from hassling with the catheter. Taking a shower was a major production. I listened to tapes from Cancer as a Turning Point and read a lot in Love, Medicine and Miracles. But the turning point for me was when I decided to put everything down and create a fresh "mind story" to repair the wall of my bladder.

In this visualization, I envisioned a gap on the floor of my bladder where the cancer had been removed. Then I watched my cells construct first a bridge across the gap, and then I saw the gap fill in. The image was very real and I attribute this to an interesting episode of Nova in which a foot bridge was being constructed across a gorge through which a river ran in the country of the Inca's somewhere in modern Peru, perhaps. The interesting thing about the Nova presentation was that the whole community turned out to build the bridge, and it was made entirely of grass ropes that everyone contributed to! So here I was, bridging the gap in my bladder with new cells constructed from grass roots of a concerted effort between all of my body resources.

When I came out of the mind story, my bag was full once again, and I felt one hundred percent better.

### 2/23/97: A Walk by the Bay

The major event of this day was a walk by the San Francisco Bay. It was a beautiful morning and I enjoyed being outdoors. However, the catheter was a drag. I had sit for a while and take my complement of deep breaths.

Later, my sister came to visit and brought smoked salmon! What a meal!

### 2/24/97: Thinking Things Over

I did not feel too well today. I had to go to Dr. Neuwirth's office today for them to take a urine sample and an hour or so later, to Dr. Slattery's office to have my teeth cleaned. While neither of them was terribly unpleasant, the combination was exhausting. At the dentist's office, I experienced teeth cleaning with ultrasound. It seemed to go faster and easier. However, I chose "laughing gas" as an escape, after which I felt a bit nauseous. At home, I took a nap and started to feel better.

Having finished *Love, Medicine & Miracles* the night before, I started reading *Cancer as a Turning Point*. It became clear to me that there are several aspects to mind-body healing. First of all, there is the necessity of a positive outlook on life and your illness. Without these, there is no place to begin. One must therefore have something to look forward to and a desire to survive. According to Dr. Siegel, in his chapter on "Becoming Exceptional," Dr. Al Siebert identifies the following indicators of self-motivated growth (and I quote):

*Aimless playfulness for its own sake, like that of a happy child.*

The ability to become so deeply absorbed in an activity that you lose track of time, external events, and all your worries, often whistling, humming or talking to yourself absentmindedly.

- A child's innocent curiosity.
- An observant, nonjudgmental style.
- Willingness to look foolish, make mistakes and laugh at yourself.
- Open-minded acceptance of criticism about yourself.
- An active imagination, daydreams, mental play, and conversations with yourself.

Dr. Siegel also identifies Al Siebert's indications of a person reaching synergistic functioning (and I quote):

Empathy for other people, including opponents.

- The ability to see patterns and relationships in organizations or equipment.

- Recognition of subliminal perception or intuition as a valid source of information.
- Good timing, especially when speaking or taking an original action.
- The ability to see early clues about future developments and take appropriate action.
- Cooperative nonconformity: refusing to be controlled by improper laws or social standards, yet choosing to abide by them most of the time for the sake of others -- unless attempting to change them. In other words, and avoidance of empty gestures.
- Being comfortable in complex, confusing situations that others find bewildering and frightening.
- Keeping a positive outlook and confidence in adversity.
- The ability to absorb new, unexpected, or unpleasant experiences and be changed by them.
- A talent for serendipity: the ability to convert what others consider accidents or misfortunes to something useful.
- The feeling of getting smarter and enjoying life more as you get older.

Although these are laudable goals, it is important for me to keep them in mind, but continue to make progress on my own. I am particularly interested in "keeping a positive outlook and confidence in adversity", as this seems to be the most difficult area for me. "Cooperative nonconformity" also sounds good to me!

In line with these observations, Dr. LeShan talks about his psychotherapeutic methods, which focus the healing energies on directing our lives towards the needs of our individual structure and what provides us with the maximum excitement in life, rather than the traditional questions of, *"What are the symptoms? What is the hidden lesion that is causing them? What can we do about the lesion, or failing that, how can we teach the person to compensate for it?"*

So really, our job as patients is to find our own true nature and not let anyone cause us to deviate from our path. This means that we have to be blatantly honest with our feelings and forget being nice, at all costs. We have to take our lives in our own hands and find out where our bliss is. We need to follow our bliss all the way to complete health and remission.

This is no small task! It requires strength and courage to confront your deepest regrets and allow them to disappear. We have to get involved so totally in our lives that we forget our illness and allow our immune system to illuminate it on its own.

## 2/25/97: A Day of Work

This morning, I resolved to fix some of the bugs that had been assigned to me. In doing so, there is often enough time to surf the web while programs are being compiled. During one such compile, I started looking for information on Dr. Stephen Sallan. He appeared on the ABC news cast last night to report on some remarkable achievements in the cure of cancer. I was really impressed with what he had to say, so I found his email address and fired off a message. The content of the message was as follows:

Dear Dr. Sallan:

I watched your presentation on ABC last night and I was really impressed. I was wondering if you wouldn't mind answering a few questions. I'll be happy to phone you if that is easier and if you provide your office number.

1. Could you please tell me the name of the agents you are using to achieve a cure? I was not able to write them down fast enough. I do remember that you use something that prevents cancer cells from constructing new blood vessels. Someone mentioned endostatin, but I thought it was after you spoke.
2. Have you done any tests with T2NoMo bladder cancer? I have been diagnosed with such and plan to have Dr. Shipley's protocol beginning on March 10. I've had two TURBTs. My guess is that you know his protocol very well. If not, I'll be happy to send it to you, or you can find it on my website (see below).
3. Does your research have anything to do with concentrated Aloe Vera or Cesium Chloride? I have heard that these naturally occurring substances have great immune building properties. Do you know anything about them?
4. Are there any trials for bladder cancer using your methods that you know of?

Thank you very much for your attention. If you have a chance, please see my web site: http://yellowstream.org. Dr. Shipley's protocol is available there.

I have found an interesting quote in *Cancer as a Turning Point* on page 95 that provides excellent support for my decision:

In contemplating the removal of an organ or organs, remember that Nature does not indulge in luxuries. As Galen wrote: "Nature does nothing in vain." If it is there, there is a good reason for it. No substitute is going to be as good (Mother Nature knows best). An organ should be removed if the alternative *at this time* is completely unacceptable. You can always have it removed later. You can't have it put back.

Other topics of interest from LeShan's book are how to survive in the hospital and how to deal with despair. He also establishes four axioms for holistic health, which I quote:

The person exists on many levels, all of which are equally real and important. Physical, psychological, and spiritual levels are one valid way of describing the person, and none of these can be "reduced" to any of the other. To move successfully towards health, all must be treated. All must be taken care of and gardened if health is to be maintained.

Each person is unique. A valid program of treatment, whether it focuses primarily on nutrition, meditation, chemotherapy, or exercise must be individualized for each person. A standardized approach to a condition is not valid under this concept.

The patient should be part of the decision making team. Each person in a program of holistic health is given as much knowledge and authority as he or she will accept.

The person has self-healing abilities. Following the first three axioms helps to mobilize these abilities and bring them to the aid of the mainline medical program.

## 2/26/97: Down with the Tube!

My catheter was finally removed this morning with such great relief. The only bad thing about the meeting with Dr. Neuwirth was that the pathology report showed that more cancer had been resected, but this doesn't change the treatment plan. We finally got the feeling the Dr. Neuwirth was behind us all the way with using the Shipley method.

We stopped by the Pine Street Clinic to pick up a powered form of the Traditional Chinese Medicinal herbs that Michael Broffman had prepared for me. Luckily, Michael was available for a brief conversation about the latest pathology report and Dr. Neuwirth's attitude. He felt strongly that it was still in my best interest to proceed with the Shipley protocol.

Later in the afternoon, I received a call from Dr. Keith Block, an internist who has put together a staff of oncologists, herbal chemists, dietitians and others who offer a combined program of chemotherapy, herbs, diet, psychological support, exercise and stress management. He is a friend of Dr. Rossman and I had placed a call to him as far back as February 9. Dr. Rossman and I had several email messages going back and forth, and finally he called back.

Dr. Block told me that he had a holistic program that attacked the cancer cells at the molecular level. He uses intervenes nutrients combined with oral agents and a detoxification program to reduce the side effects of the chemotherapy. He uses fractional dosages for optimum effectiveness combined with patient comfort. The rest of his life-affirming program consists of nutrition, exercise, supplements and stress management techniques.

I really felt confused after speaking with him, as he likes to treat patients in his facility in Evanston, IL. While it is not out of the question for me to travel to Evanston (after all, I spent three years of my life in Chicago and three years of my life in Evanston!), I would be giving up all my support systems back in the Bay Area. So after an excellent guided imagery session with Leslie Davenport, a very supportive conversation with Dr. Rossman, and a good night's sleep, I felt better about staying with the plan I already had in place.

# 5 - ACCELERATED GROWTH

## 2/27/97: Cancerport

Cancer Port is a support group that meets on Thursdays from 11:30 A. M. until 1:00 P. M. in Greenbrae. The purpose of the group is the emotional support of its members, which varies from time to time. On this particular occasion, there were approximately twenty-five men and women with various types of cancer, including several support people and three group facilitators. There were no other people with bladder cancer in the group.

When it became my turn to talk, I explained how I was diagnosed and what sort of treatment I was about to undergo. I talked about my fears of still having cancer eight weeks after the start of chemotherapy. Seeing what other people suffered with made me feel compassionate for their situations and increased my desire to share the research I had been doing since my diagnosis.

I left the meeting with two important things to do based on what people said. One of them was to contact Dr. Shipley to find out what the side effects of the cisplatin and 5-FU were, and how to counteract them. The other was to make an appointment with Dr. Van Vu for next Sunday. I felt under a lot of stress until these could be accomplished. Instead of breathing into the experience of tension, I drove home, had lunch and only after I made the phone calls did I feel any better.

Later in the afternoon I had an appointment with Dr. Barbara Rose Billings, a special healer who provides "Integration Therapy" which is a "multi-faceted and individualized to help give you what you need to unleash the healing power within you. Its strength lies in its ability to produce profound results by integrating your essence into the healing process." I had an extremely healing experience with her, in recognizing what I want to do, tuning into my "belly breath", and being recognized for my own healing abilities.

## 2:/28/97: The Papilla Tree in the Forest

Early this morning, I received a call back from Dr. Shipley, and I asked him about the side effects of the chemotherapy and radiation. He said that I should have a positive attitude and perhaps I'd feel a little tired, but I shouldn't worry! I guess he knows! This set me up for a fine day!

I next attended Leslie Davenports cancer group at Marin General Hospital. During the guided imagery, I was taken by two images that were very healing. The first was an emotionally open heart that reminded me of Ram Dass' song:

> Listen, listen, listen to my heart's song...
> I will never forget you, I will never forsake you.
> Listen, listen, listen to my heart's song...
> I will never forget you, I will never forsake you.

The second image was even more powerful. There I was, sitting under the papilla tree with Siddhartha Gautama, and I realized that he was sitting there for me. It was now up to me to sit under the tree for those that follow me. It was a powerful image that connected me directly to the Buddha and his teachings of emptiness and the path with a heart. On completion of the guided imagery, I drew a picture, on which I wrote,

> The Buddha sat under the papaya tree for me...
> I must sit under it for those that follow me.

### 3/1/97: A Day with Friends and Family

Today was spent almost entirely with friends and family. In the morning, we were visited by Dr. John Anderson and family, who had spent the previous night. They are from Nashville, TN, but love to drop in on us in Sausalito. We had a nice leisurely walk by the bay and talked of many things. Later, my cousins came over from Oakland.

All of this made me fairly exhausted, so I listened to a guided imagery tape preparing me for chemotherapy. I found the tape to be confusing because the speaker offered too many choices. I find that following specific directions is much more useful than something like, "Pick a relaxing spot - maybe a beach, or a meadow, or a mountain top, or..." I seem to pick all of the places as they are mentioned and wind up picking none. However, once I adjusted to the changing scenery, I relaxed quite nicely and utilized the tape to develop a sense of what good the chemotherapy would do for me.

At night, we visited our friends who had been on a trip to Africa and viewed their collection of slides. I was impressed with the quality of their photographs and their caring support. Besides, the food was great.

All in all, it was a pleasant day almost entirely removed from thoughts of my illness. Sometimes it's good to allow your illness to float to the background and have a normal life. This gives you a hint of what life will be like when the disease goes into remission.

### 3/2/97: Qi Gong

My friend, Itzzy, came over today to teach me qi gong once again. He had taught me several years ago, but I wanted a new lesson because of Michael Broffman's recommendation. Itzzy has been practicing and teaching tai chi and qi gong for almost twenty years. His teach is Fong Ha.

We started with sitting meditation. It turned out to be very closely related to the Vipassana meditation that I was already doing, except for the emphasis on the out breath. The posture is upright with the buttocks on the edge of the chair and the spine erect. The hands are either placed on the knees with the thumb and forefingers making a "U" and facing each other, or interlocked in front of the point between the navel and the pubic bone (the *da tien* point in *qi gong* or *hara* in Zen). The process is to watch the breath fill up a balloon in the lower abdomen and return to the breath whenever the mind wanders away.

The second form is standing meditation. Here, the breath and attention work the same from a standing position. The feet are parallel and shoulder width apart, and the hands are either at the side, or somewhere in an arc from the *da tien* point to the throat, where ever the optimum comfort and/or awareness lies. We tried various configurations, all of which seemed to work quite well.

The next thing we tried was walking meditation, which is similar to walking meditation in Vipassana, except the feet are swung in a slight semi-circle from one placement to another. Finally, we did some rocking meditation, which is very comforting when you feel that you have to move a little more.

I loved being with Itzzy and being shown these various postures. We walked a while and then had pizza at my house.

After Itzzy left, I listened to another guided imagery tape and later started *Practical Intuition* by Laura Day. I was lucky to have met Laura at Eselan when I was invited there by Helen Palmer for an organizational meeting of the *Center for Investigation and Training of the Intuition* in 1988. Her book is a marvelous training guide and I plan to utilize it as much as possible in my healing.

### 3/3/97: Healing the Body - Healing the Mind

The morning started out with a Feldenkrais class incorporating arm movements. I couldn't believe how exhausted I was when returned home! I found it necessary to settle into another guided imagery tape after lunch to even have a chance of making my day.

Next came a very revealing guided imagery session with Leslie Davenport at Marin General. I began talking about my fears of the upcoming chemotherapy and radiation and traced the fears down many, many levels to my fears of abandonment and treatment with indifference that experienced as a child. While there wasn't time for a complete resolution of the situation, I think that there is much more work to do in this area. I feel rather pressured to perform because I have expectations of completing the Shipley protocol with a complete response and not have remaining cancer at the end of April or the beginning of May when my next TURBT will be.

After this session, I took a thirty minute walk on the pathway near the hospital to absorb what I had learned from my meditation and to allow the images to integrate into my life. As I was walking back to my car, I had this wonderful feeling of making myself lovable, not only to myself, but to everyone I saw and came in contact with. I took this feeling into Anna Halprin's group and it turned into one of the most healing events of my life. I was open to receiving and giving love and there was plenty to go around! We had a large discussion on alternative healing prior to our movement program.

The movement program focused on prayer, and I don't know if Anna picked up this idea from me, or I got it several minutes before she said anything, but it was the exact word I would have chosen! This intuitive flash led to an immensely moving dance, which brought the whole group together in one circle, filled with healing energy and love.

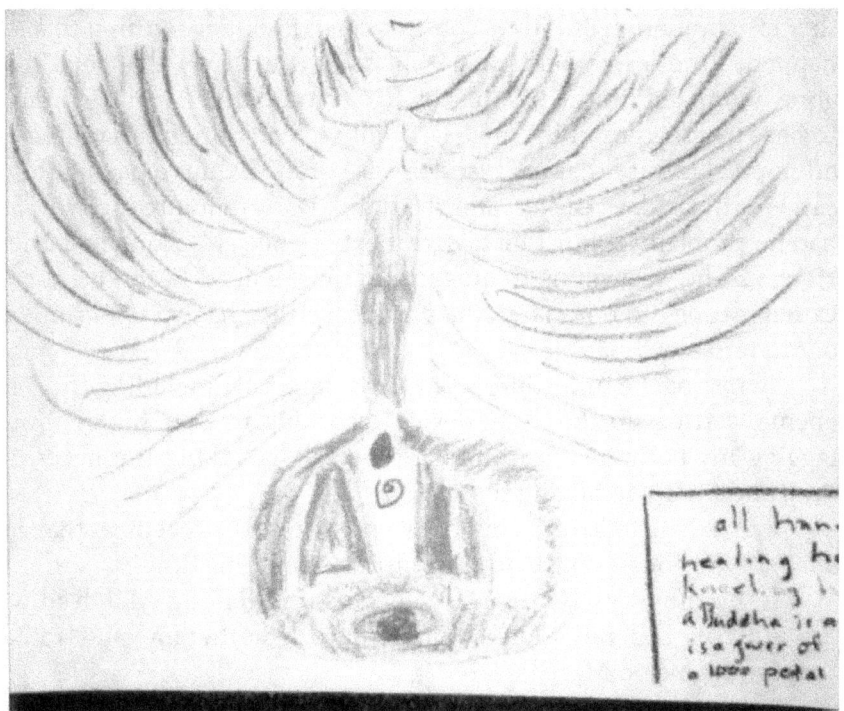

I drew a picture of myself kneeling in the prayer position with my hands drawn together in the traditional prayer position. The hands were way out of proportion, but as the drawing developed, I began to realize that I was also drawing the healing space around my hand and the healing energy radiating from them. I wrote,

*all hands*
*healing hands*
*kneeling hands*
*a Buddha is a rose is a giver of qi*
*a 1000 petal lotus*

Something remarkable is taking place as I focus on healing my cancer. I find that I can't but help heal my whole self. Without healing my whole self, there can be no healing of my cancer. They are strongly interconnected as all phenomena of the universe are. And, I believe, this is the essence of holistic health - healing the body and healing the mind. This is what I'm striving for and what I want to achieve.

## 3/4/97: "Humor Comes a Year Later"

The above quote was Dr. Halberg's comment as we left the radiation therapy simulation session. "You will laugh about everything that happened today in about a year!" she said. Everything that could have gone wrong did! In the first place I had to walk to Dr. Neuwirth's office to have a catheter put in, since Dr. Halberg had difficulties on two attempts. I'm sure that my bladder was sensitive due to having the catheter in six days earlier, and she didn't want to injure me. But, Harry had no problem! It must be his great experience at putting in catheters! However, he was willing to hurt me, but just a little. Secondly, the catheter tube did not match the syringe, so they had to send someone out to find a compatible syringe.

The rest of the procedure went fairly smoothly including the Barium enema, setting up the x-ray device according to the Shipley protocol, tagging my body for future radiation sessions, taking the necessary x-rays, and finally removing the tubing.

I was exhausted from this hour and one half procedure that lasted almost four hours! I have nothing else to say at this time!

Oh, by the way, the treatment begins on Monday, March 10 with a dry run on the radiation equipment. Chemotherapy and radiation therapy begins on March 11.

### 3/5/97: Another CT Scan

Last night, I watched a series of programs on public television featuring Dr. Andrew Weil. I have transcribed my notes as part of this diary (see http://yellowstream.org/drweil.htm). Please take a look if you are interested.

This morning, I had another CT scan for the purpose of setting up the radiation fields that I will be using next week. Alice, the radiation technologist made everything so easy. She was easy going, gentle, and caring. I felt fortunate that I was treated so nicely.

The rest of the day was spent working, having teacher conferences, doing guided imagery, and catching up on things. I have also started reading *Practical Intuition* and doing all of the exercises.

### 3/6/97: "I'm Amazed at How Well the Body Can Heal Itself"

Last night, I felt a little anxious as I went to bed. I felt that I hadn't done enough for my treatment during the day and needed some more time to work on myself. I came downstairs to listen to a tape by Dr. Bernie Siegel called Meditations for Enhancing Your Immune System.

After listening to the tape for 25 minutes or so, I found myself moved to tears. It was the first time I had really cried since the beginning of this episode. I couldn't get a fix on what made me cry or why I was crying. The whole thing is just so emotional that you can't help but be moved.

I attended another Cancerport group this morning, but I didn't have much to say about my own situation. However, I did advise one young man to seek alternative therapies as a way of enhances his chances of recovery. I told another man about my son's kidney cancer and he seemed hopeful. All in all, it was a good group and I felt at peace.

In the afternoon, I took a walk and stopped by to see D. S., who has been battling ovarian cancer since 1991. She told me about her treatments and had one major comment that we should all be aware of, "I am amazed at how well the body can heal itself!"

That night, we had a meeting of our evolutionary circle at T. W.'s house. R. and J. did not make it, but this did not detract from the value of the meeting. B. M. and T. W. both got to speak their truth and I spent a lot of time sharing what was has been happening with me. I described all of the healers I've been seeing and told them about some of my best experiences. T. W. had oral cancer, from which she is recovered, and she is also writing a book about her experiences, and how cancer changed her life. She read her preface, which was very helpful for me.

### 3/7/97: La Boheme

Today I have a busy schedule. I see Dr. Gullion in the morning, meet with co-workers in the early afternoon, and travel to Capitola for my son's performance in La Boheme in the evening. We have planned to spend the night in Capitola. I have prepared a list of questions for Dr. Gullion.

Once again, Dr. Gullion showed up with a heart pin on his shirt pocket. I believe that he is quite open to what Andy Weil calls *integrative medicine*. We spoke about all the issues on the list and the thing that struck me the most was his willingness to allow guided imagery and massage along with chemotherapy. He said that this is what they were trying to do at the Marin Cancer Institute.

As far as Keith Block is concerned, Dr. Gullion thought that with Michael Broffman and all that I was doing, it amounts to the same thing. He said that he had always had difficulty getting Dr. Block to be specific about what he is doing, and that he had proprietary supplement preparations that no one else had. I felt confident that I was on the right path because of Michael Broffman, Marty Rossman, Van Vu, Elyse, and the combination of all the other things I am doing.

As far as the chemotherapy is concerned, he was no more worried about my response than Dr. Shipley. He had given cisplatin and 5FU together before, but not combined with radiation and not in the doses that I will be getting.

After our visit with Dr. Gullion, we headed down to Network General and then to Santa Cruz. We checked in to the Apple Lane Inn and took a nap before meeting M. and G. for dinner in Capitola before the opera. M. seemed quite relaxed in spite of having one of the leading roles in the production. I was feeling quite proud of him and also felt excited to be able to be there. You may recall that on my first visit to Dr. Neuwirth's office when he described my illness, I wanted to be able to see La Boheme.

The performance was rather good for the first performance of a new opera company. Of course my son had the best male performance as Marcello, Rudolpho's friend! The woman who played Mussetta was also excellent. But the orchestra and chorus left something to be desired. All in all, it was very enjoyable and I recommend it to anyone living near Santa Cruz.

### 3/8/97: A Day of Traveling

Last night was a difficult night for me as far as sleep is concerned. I kept sliding into the middle of the bed and woke up frequently. Then the roosters started crowing early in the morning.

We walked along the Santa Cruz Beach Boardwalk for about an hour and then headed for Los Gatos. We thought we'd have lunch there, but wound up being tourists. We had dinner at the Rossman's and I went to the Pocket Opera performance of *Escape from the Harem*. All in all, it was a busy day without too much concern about cancer.

### 3/9/97: A Nice Day by the Bay

We had to go to a first communion ceremony this morning, and for me, this is an unusual experience. There were several interesting things about the service. First of all, there were many prayers that I remember from my youth in synagogue. Although I knew this to be true from before, it really struck home today because of my acute awareness of little things in life due to my illness. I almost felt like belting out the Hebrew for the prayers!

Secondly, I was reminded of one of my favorite prayers growing up. It goes like this:

*May the words of my mouth*
*and the meditations of my heart*
*Be acceptable to Thee*
*in Thy sight Oh Lord,*
*My strength and my redeemer.*

I recited this prayer along with the Shemah each night before I went to bed. Now I observe my breath and do other breathing exercises. As long as each is done with spirit, they have the possibility of achieving the same result of peace of mind and a wise and understanding heart which can discern between good and evil.

The views from the church were the first occurrence of spectacular views of the day.

I left early to meet my friends from my enneagram circle group who met me at home. We went on down to Sausalito, and enjoyed a nice lunch at a picnic table by the bay. We spoke of treatment options and alternative medicine. I felt totally supported by my friends.

Unfortunately, I had to leave them for an acupuncture treatment with Dr. Van Vu, which was quite relaxing. Instead of going home and resting, I drove to Belvedere to take a walk with T. R We saw panoramic views of San Francisco, Oakland and the East Bay, and of course, Sausalito! What a gorgeous day! It makes you want to be alive, just to feel the clean, fresh air flowing through your lungs. Boy, was I exhausted, though.

## 3/10/97: King of the Jungle of the Mind

This morning, I had to go back to Radiation Oncology department to have a dry run of my radiation treatments. This went rather smoothly, but I noticed that the waiting room was filled with older people! I thought, "I'm too young to have cancer!" This thought doesn't seem to do me any good!

While I was waiting, I continued reading in *Practical Intuition*. One of the experiments was to open yourself to your sense impressions according to the instructions,

"To begin, simply start reporting what you're sensing in the moment. If you hear a car beeping outside, say so. If your nose itches, say so (feel free to scratch it). If you're hungry, say so. The trick is to report everything you notice-out loud. Don't forget to report any thoughts, feelings, or memories that you become aware of." - From *Practical Intuition*, by Laura Day, page 54.

I wrote down my impressions and then I was called in for the dry run. After that, I decided to take a walk along the beautiful stream that flows into the bay across from Marin General Hospital. I had chosen to walk at least two miles. As I walked, I noticed the birds, flowers and other plants, and especially Mount Tamalpais. Before I reached the mile mark to turn around, I noticed that I was behind 919 Sir Francis Drake, where I had my company in 1982. I decided to continue on to Willie's Caffe and have breakfast, but I didn't have any money. I only brought my car key, the stone from Anna Halprin, and the ammonite fossil that Barbara Rose Billings had given me. So I asked the manager if I could give her a credit card number. She said no, but would feed me anyway on an "IOU!" Well, I really enjoyed my pancakes, poached eggs, and bacon, with a large glass of fresh orange juice!

As I was leaving the restaurant, I spotted two angels across the street: J. D. and her friend, M. J. J. D. is the mother of my daughter's best friend. I asked J. if she had some money, and her friend had $14.00 that she had discovered after she got out of the car. Normally, neither one of them would have money with them, but on this occasion, she had just the amount I needed! So I borrowed the money from M. and paid my bill. Not only that, but J. and M. were walking back to Marin General Hospital to get their car with their dogs, so I joined them and we enjoyed a marvelous hike back to the cars!

One of the plans for today was to prepare for the chemo and radiation therapy tomorrow. In accordance with this plan, Dr. Gullion had given me a list of suggestions. One of them corresponds to exactly what the Shipley protocol demands: patient hydration of 3 to 4 quarts of fluids. So that's what I spent the afternoon doing!

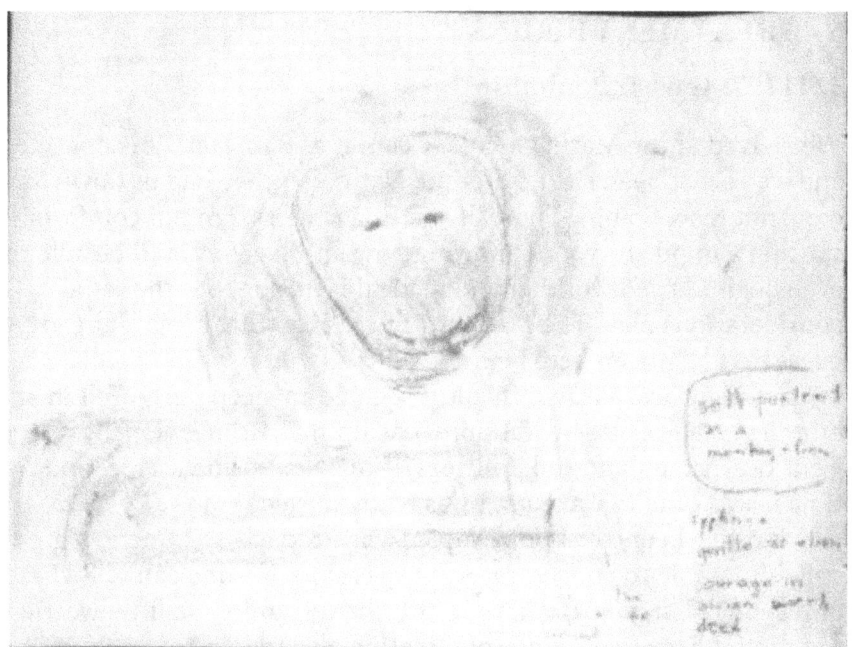

Since it was Monday night, I went to Anna Halprin's class. Again, it was absolutely healing. The themes for the night were deep breathing and choosing an animal to represent our condition or needs. The deep breathing was inspired by Andy Weil. For my animal, I chose a lion, an image I had had about a year ago. In fact, the wallpaper for my computer at work is a picture of a lion, and of all the animals at P. G.'s house, I was most attracted to the lions. We drew pictures of our animals and then danced the pictures. The picture I drew reminded me of a Sphinx. It looked like a self-portrait of a monkey-lion. The major theme was the courage I need to endure the next eight weeks, and the significance of the Sphinx was the guardian of the temple so that only those with a pure heart could enter. The spirit of the lion I chose was one of a contented cat who was rolled over on his back and relaxing.

The class ended with a healing circle. Anna placed me in the center so that I could receive the energy of the group for my treatments tomorrow. It was very powerful!

## 6 - TREATMENT BEGINS

### 3/11/97: Jewish Penicillin

We arrived at the Marin Oncology center at 8:10. Here it is now 9:03 and we've just been sitting around. Naturally, they had us down for 9:00, not 8:00. So now I'm really getting restless. I'm not comfortable starting a mind story, not knowing how far I'll get or if I'll be able to even begin. I tried working on Practical Intuition, but the same considerations play. The man next to me is getting his i. v. already. I guess that he's been here before.

Last night was fairly difficult. I seemed to sleep fairly well in stages, but due to all of the hydration, I was up many times. Finally, at 3:00, I went downstairs and did a little writing. Next came a tape, and by the time it was time to wake up, I was ready to sleep.

I haven't been that preoccupied with today's treatment plan, but I still felt unable to concentrate on my breath. No one can tell what kind of response I'm going to have to the chemo, and I'm a little worried. To top it off, I have two rounds of radiation also today.

I had expected to be able to listen to guided imagery tapes, but with all the commotion going around here, I preferred to listen to the classical CD's I brought. The Beethoven *Choral Fantasy* brought on a lot of emotion. I also listened to Dvorak's *Piano Quintet* and Shubert's *Trout Quintet*. These pieces of music are so calming and beautiful. I use my computer as my portable CD player.

Once the 5FU and cisplatin where into my blood stream, I felt a few minor discomforts, but all in all, it wasn't too bad - just like Shipley predicted. I can probably have a decent afternoon. As soon as the cisplatin was finished, I got an urge for matzoth ball soup from Max's! When I was growing up, this was called, "Jewish penicillin!"

I started having pains in my stomach and needed to pee again! The pains didn't last long and I continued to pee frequently. At around 1:15 P. M., an hour and a half after the cisplatin was totally in, I went down for my first radiation treatment. Although I was a little nervous, I came through it OK. Within the next half-hour, we were back upstairs, getting the i. v. out and on our way home. Although I felt very tired, there were no other side effects. I was advised to take a sedative tonight to get some sleep, but now that the unknown is known, will I need it?

The second radiation treatment went really well. I was able to be relaxed and visualize the radiation helping the cancer cells to mutate back to healthy cells normal cells, or, if they choose, to self-destruct. This seemed to be really effective. The radiologist placed tattoos for the spots for focusing the beam and then explained the computerized care that I was getting.

## 3/12/97: Chopped Liver

The night before last I couldn't sleep because of the anxiety over the unknown effects of chemotherapy and radiation. Last night I couldn't sleep because I was waiting for side effects, which didn't come! So today, I really exhausted. I hope to get my energy up by the time we leave.

I spent the time listening to guided imagery tapes, Deepak Chopra, and surfing the news groups on the web. I had an interesting query from a reader of the news group, alt.support.cancer.

The second day of 5FU and cisplatin was similar to the first. This time I had a chopped chicken liver sandwich for lunch from Max's! It went well again, although I fell a little exhausted.

After the chemotherapy, I had another guided imagery session with Leslie Davenport. The session was interrupted by an extremely urgent need to pee. Before then, I was visualizing how the chemotherapy and radiation were helping me either revert the cancer cells back to normal cells, or at their choice, bubble up and degenerate into something that could be easily eliminated by the blood stream, urine, and feces. I got some really good images to work with in the future.

We stopped by M. C.'s house to see the girls before the fly off to Palm Springs for the weekend while I recover from my three doses of chemotherapy and four doses of radiation.

I spent a lot of time trying to fix a bug (work for money), so there's not much more to say. The fact that I feel like fixing is actually saying a lot.

## 3/13/97: Hair Raising Experience

Compared to yesterday, I'm not feeling as well, even though I appeared to have more sleep. I feel a little nauseous and a bit constipated. I also feel rather tired. I think I did too much work yesterday, and I continue to work even as I write this, being interrupted by break points in my code. After a while I couldn't code anymore and decided to sit back and listen to a tape of Deepak Chopra. I must have dozed off a couple of times during the tape, because before I knew it, I was finished with the cisplatin.

When I got home after the first round of radiation for the day, I could do nothing but crash. I focused in on my breath in my belly, and before I knew it, I had a nice nap, only to be awakened by having to pee. I tried to accomplish some work, but felt quite queasy.

Then it was time to go for the second radiation treatment. I felt the hair on my body rise as the radiation impacted my body. This distracted me slightly from my visualization of the cancer cells shriveling up and being properly eliminated. I really felt badly the rest of the day and into the night.

### 3/14/97: One Day at a Time

Things are now in motion for the first rounds of chemoradiotherapy to work. The elimination state begins and I feel fair to middling this morning. I'm going to try to do some symbolic cleaning up in my office once I get some more bugs fixed and then try to make Leslie Davenport's class.

Leslie's class was taught by an art therapist this time and we built worry dolls. My doll was named Homer and he has to worry about the next TURBT revealing no cancer!

After a nice lunch, I crashed for an hour and a half.

### 3/16/97: Raining in California

I wasn't able to write anything yesterday. I felt really lousy. I needed a lot of rest and spent some of the day with company. I was feeling a bit nauseous all day and didn't feel too much like eating, even though my wife made smoked salmon caviar pizza! It was a day to vege out and forget about cancer. Maybe that's good to do once in a while!

### 3/17/97: Cancer Sucks!

During the past two days, I have noticed many instances of random tears. Most of the time, they seem to come from nowhere, but other times, I am aware of what triggered them. For example, we watched two pre-recorded episodes of Nova last night which dealt with cancer. Most of the people on the shows were in much worse shape than I, and I felt compassion for their suffering. I realized that it was also my suffering and I wanted my life back. Another example: today, my daughter's best friend's mother had a lumpectomy, and I felt badly for her. Much of the time, I simply feel the tragedy of the disease.

Other than these random acts of crying, I've had a pretty productive day. I did an adequate job at work, and although I felt nauseous most of the day, I managed to get by. Naturally, my afternoon "mind story" was quite helpful, both in calming my nausea and allowing me to relax and visualize the cancer shrinking.

### 3/18/97: A Walk by the Bay

Today was the best day I had so far since the chemotherapy and radiation! I spent a lot of time working today, but at noon I took a long break. I took a walk in Sausalito by the San Francisco Bay, where all the tourists come. The walk was especially nice, since I felt well enough to do it! After walking all the way from the center of town to the Chart House restaurant, I stopped at a beautiful spot near the end of the walkway that is closest to the water. There is a place there where the concrete ends and a gravel path of about 25 feet begins. It has a lovely view of the Bay, Angel Island, and San Francisco. I stopped there to do some stretches and qi gong. The weather was magnificent and it really felt good to be out on my own again. Hopefully, I'll do something similar to this tomorrow!

I found myself drinking much more today, as this helps to hydrate my system and eliminate the dead cancer cells. This was the first day that I could manage this. I am now in the process of preparing my system for the next phase of chemotherapy and radiation on Tuesday, March 25. I'll keep you posted!

### 3/19/97: Massage and Tennis

Today was another wonderful day! I had a massage at the Marin Oncology Center from Nora O'Toole, a Certified Massage Therapist who donates her time and energy to work with patients. This is also a part of the Marin General Hospital Humanities Program, along with the guided imagery sessions I've been having with Leslie Davenport.

After the massage, I couldn't help but drive by Boyle Park to see whether I could play some tennis. I sat for a while, amazed at the empty courts, and rubbed sun block over the exposed parts of my body just in case the 5FU was still active. I was feeling so normal that when the opportunity to hit with someone came along, I took the opportunity! Man, was it fun! I found myself hitting the ball with the out breath, just as planned, but not consciously thought of. I played only for about forty-five minutes, but it felt great!

On the way home, I bought a new tennis racket to celebrate my recovery. After trying out several rackets, I settled on a Prince because it felt intuitively correct for me. This was a direct experience from my study of *Practical Intuition*.

Later on in the day, I received a call from Jeff Barber, a Reiki practitioner. He was given my name by a friend of ours who utilized his healing abilities for serious burns suffered by their daughter as a result of an automobile accident. They reported wonderful things about Reiki and I wanted to find out how it could help me. Since Jeff also has a home in Lake Tahoe, I wasn't able to speak with him until today. I have a feeling that the Reiki method is not to different from many of the healing techniques I use with my children.

In addition to telling me about his Zen practice and his exposure to the teachings of some wonderful Tibetan Buddhists, he told me about a medical doctor who had people write about the reasons for their illness in pencil. Specifically, he suggested writing a letter to "Dear Cancer in My Body." In the letter, you write emotionally about all the things that are bothering you about your illness, especially your anger, irritation, concerns, broken dreams and promises. You are to release all of these things thorough this writing. It should be done in pencil with your own hand writing and later burned with or without ceremony.

The theory behind this lies in the three carbon factors involved: the human body, the pencil (graphite), and the paper, which turns into carbon when burned. He has seen and heard about people walking away from all kinds of physical and emotional distress. Through the process of writing, the incident you're writing about becomes complete, and you are not holding on to it anymore physically, emotionally, or spiritually. This transmutation of emotion that led to the illness seems to work wonders.

When writing, release all the anger, irritation, broken dreams, promises, and other negative emotions that you have ever felt, as the illness could have be caused by factors in your childhood, and taken decades to develop physically. Release all of this through the writing and burning. The process lets you come more into the present because you are not bringing any of the past into the present. Write about every hard moment in your life and release the emotional charge so that it no longer has a hold on physical body. When writing to the cancer in your body, state that you're releasing the cancer from your body and there's no place for it and there is no longer any benefit from it. State that you don't need the cancer to bring you in to the present moment. Write about anything that bugs you. Write to the fact that you are taking chemotherapy and radiation and they're not going to have effects that the body doesn't want. Remind yourself that you don't have to buy into the results of the allopathic medical doctors.

In the end, he recommended the book, *Reclaiming Your Health - Breaking the Medical Myth* by John Robbins, heir to the Baskin-Robbins fortune, which he gave up because he didn't believe that ice cream (as good as it is!) is good for your health!

I am definitely looking forward to meeting Jeff Barber!

### 3/20/97: Tennis, Cancerport, and Feldenkrais

Today was an up and down day, with the highs being much greater than the lows. In the morning, I was experiencing some of the side effects from radiation therapy resulting in diarrhea. Even so, I managed to play two sets of tennis with some of my favorite players. Naturally, I had no symptoms while I was on the court!

Later in the morning, I took my wife to Cancerport with me. It was really nice to have her there and experience the people I have become attached to, simply because we share similar life circumstance. I mainly shared my experience of the chemotherapy and radiation, and that I was feeling well enough to play tennis. All three of the leaders commented on how therapeutic tennis could be and I agreed with them by stating that I'd prefer to play tennis than attend a support group. So it is likely that I'll miss Leslie Davenport's group tomorrow because I'm scheduled to play tennis at 8:30 in the morning on the *first day of spring*!

From Cancerport, I went to get my new racket strung and then to G. T.'s for a Feldenkrais lesson. It was truly amazing! She was so attuned to my body that she discovered my traditional places of where I hold tension. Not only that, but I experienced the transmission of energy through my skeletal system as she pressed and manipulated various areas. The climax was when she rolled me up to a sitting position! This was quite remarkable, as one moment I was lying on my side and the next moment I was sitting up, and the transition was made so seamlessly that I felt totally reassured, comfortable, and relaxed. I highly recommend stopping by to have a session with Gail!

When I finally got home, I picked up the mail and became stressed out even before I opened it! I had stressful items to deal with from the IRS, the State Board of Equalization, and Cigna Health Care. The stress I felt was in addition to being exhausted from all my activities. Nevertheless, I proceeded to do a mind story, and felt a little relieved. Then I realized that the best way to deal with the stressful items was simply to tackle them one at a time.

## 3/21/97: It's All Downhill From Here

Once again, I spent the morning playing tennis. It was very nice to play with J., V., and C. These are some of my favorite partners and we all get along so well. On the court next to us was another foursome that I often play with. D. F. and E. M. even visited me in the hospital during the second TURBT. I felt comfortable and excited to have the opportunity to play again.

C. was having a tough time getting into her game. She had not been playing much lately, because of work obligations, so her game was a little off. I coached her to remain anchored in her body and focus on her belly breath. From then on, her game improved. Nevertheless, we all had a marvelous time!

I had a conversation with my son in which he told me about two productions that he could play in. One is a Victor Herbert production of *Naughty Marietta*. The other is *The Barber of Seville*, with the same production company that produced *La Boheme*. He was telling me that the lead role in *The Barber of Seville* may be too difficult for him and maybe he should settle for a more limited role. He seems to be quite confused about this matter. So, being a good dad, I expressed to him how I thought that the people who succeed in the entertainment business really stretch themselves and go for the top productions that they can get in to. He is taking my advice under consideration.

In the afternoon I had the best guided imagery session that I ever had with Leslie Davenport! After talking a while about the details of my recovery, I decided to simply see what came up for me in the session, rather than have a planned agenda. The session was so incredible that I decided to incorporate a large portion of it in the transcript on the

*Mindfulness in Healing* website (see http://www.mindfulnessinhealing.org/guided-imagery-transcript). It really speaks for itself, and I invite you to explore it!

### 3/22/97: Visiting J. B.

The first thing I did this morning was to fire off an email message to John Gray. Hopefully, he'll write back or phone me. His daughter will be in middle school with mine next year!

I spent a large part of the morning and early afternoon working on the Sniffer and making copies of video tapes. I have mentioned that I had viewed two Nova episodes that we recorded sometime last week, and a lady at Cancerport on Thursday wanted to see them. I also made several copies of the **In Search of ... Faith Healing** that my son appeared on to distribute to the various cancer support libraries around the county. My son will convert segment about him to a *Quicktime* movie and I'll post it on this web site as soon as it becomes available.

One of the nicest things to happen today was my visit with J. B. She had surgery last Monday and is doing fine. However, a friend of hers is having difficulty with lung cancer and J, feels that she would benefit from guided imagery. I offered to train her and J. thought this would really work out fine for her friend financially. So, we'll see what happens when I re-launch my career as a guided imagery teacher! J. also gave me updated wallet photos of Meher Baba, who originated the affirmation, "Don't worry, be happy!" I have carried one of these cards in my wallet for the last twenty-five to thirty years. Her husband makes annual journeys to India to visit his ashram.

### 3/23/97: Lunch at Mikayla's

After a couple of hours of tennis with the guys at Edgewood Park, I had lunch at Mikayla's with J. M., his daughter and C. H. C. H. is an author, lecturer, and business consultant. He is also on the Board of Directors for Future Medicine. He told J. and I about magnetic field therapy, which we plan to look into in greater detail. Apparently, there are two choices for this therapy: travel to the Dominican Republic, pay $20,000 for a guaranteed cure. The other is to meet a man from Utah somewhere in Canada or Mexico and pay only his expenses to have a similar treatment. I'll keep you posted when I find out more information.

C. also advised me to keep the book simple and not give too much advice! In conjunction with this, he mentioned the following items:

Take 1 TBS. of fresh flax seed oil per 100 pounds of body weight with sulphureted proteins obtainable from yogurt, milk, and certain vegetables. This method is espoused by Dr. Johanna Budwig. Also, Dr. Mary Enig in this country speaks about the same thing.

For people of Northern European descent needs to take gamma-linoleic acid 2000 mg twice a day. This can be found in evening primrose oil.

There is some new research on rice bran to hit the wires soon!

Later that evening, we went to our friend's house for dinner on Mount Tamalpais and watched the eclipse of the moon. The views from their house were awe inspiring!

## 3/24/97: Healthy Cells Grow All By Themselves

I passed up an opportunity to play tennis today because I didn't want to be too exhausted for my chemotherapy and radiation therapy tomorrow. We still need a fourth and I wasn't about to play singles. So I spent most of the day working except for a two hour break to visit on of the members of Cancerport who hadn't be showing up and who sent her husband as an emissary. The visit was something I felt I could do for the lady and I also wanted her to know about Aloe Vera and Cesium Chloride treatments.

Speaking of cesium chloride, I had a rather long conversation with Michael Broffman about the meeting with C. H. and especially about the strategy for what we were going to do after Thursday. Cesium chloride seems like a good possibility.

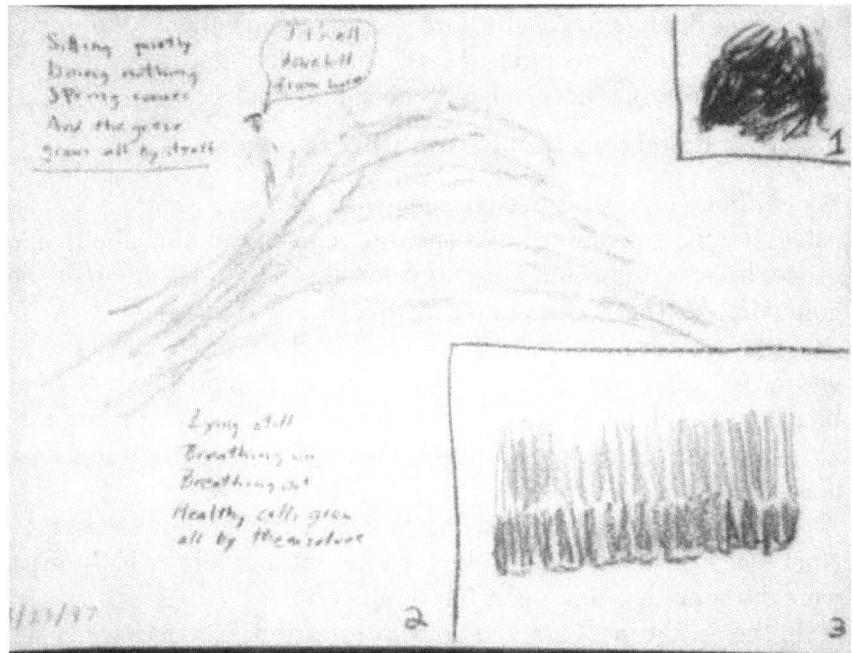

At night, I went to Anna Halprin's class only to find that she wasn't there. The class was taught very capably by two of her students, and I felt tremendous joy as I shared my experience with Leslie Davenport on Friday. I felt totally loved and supported. I danced and drew the experience. In the drawing, I wrote,

> Lying still,
> Breathing in, Breathing out,
> Healthy cells grow all by themselves!
> I am free of cancer!

Naturally, this was based on the Zen poem previously mentioned.

### 3/25/97: More Chemotherapy, More Radiation

The second round of chemotherapy and radiation therapy began today. Aside from being a little late, it went quite smoothly. I especially enjoyed the visits of K. S. and Leslie Davenport. I spoke to Leslie about working with her doing guided imagery through the Humanities Program and Marin General Hospital. She suggested that I offer my services over the web. Watch for a new topic on services!

D. B. took me to my second radiotherapy of the day. We had a nice conversation about our common interests and she bought me a book by Sylvia Boorstein, That's Funny, You Don't Look Buddhist. I'm looking forward to reading it! As you probably know by now, I am a living example of a Jubu - a Jewish born Buddhist.

## 3/26/97: Bagel and Lox Cream Cheese Spread

My mother would have been 81 today had she not died of an osteosarcoma almost ten years ago. I have been thinking about all the cancer in our family, and it is really outrageous. Something must be going on here that we have no control over.

Today's treatment went more quickly than yesterday's, and lunch was great! All I needed to feel quite good by 6:00 PM was a guided imagery tape of Leslie Davenport and a short nap. My wife and the kids have been very supportive, and I expect to fly through these days quite well.

While the cisplatin was being infused I had another massage with Nora. Because of the IV, and the time limitations, all she had time to do were my shoulders and neck, but it felt good.

In the meantime, I worked on the professional services web page.

I have decided to photograph the drawings I've done at Anna Halprin's classes. One of them was linked into the day before yesterday.

## 3/27/97: The Last Day of Treatment

Today's treatment was the most difficult for me of all. I was tired from the very beginning and thank God I had good tapes to listen to drown out the ambient noise in the room. A. M. and R. M. came to visit me at the oncology center, and they brought cheerfulness and smart conversation with them.

I came home and went right to sleep (after checking email)! I used Leslie Davenport's tape and it worked quite well. T. R. is picking me up in a few minutes for the last of the radiation treatments.

I started reading *That's Funny, You Don't Look Buddhist* last night and fired off an email to her. I'm looking forward to what she has to say, and I'd even like to have a session with her.

I also fired off an email message to the Zero Balancing page, and it was forwarded to Fritz Smith. I already heard from Fritz and he had a lot of nice things to say!

So now that I've done all of this writing, I'm feeling a little better. Each time I get low on energy, I have to resort to "breathing in I'm healing myself, breathing out I'm clear of cancer," or, more shortly, in the spirit of Thich Nhat Hanh, "healing... clear... healing... clear... "

## 7 - WAITING FOR A COMPLETE RESPONSE

### 3/28/97: "Waiting is ... Grocking in Fullness"

Today we begin the long wait for the results of the induction chemotherapy and radiation therapy. Frankly, I am quite pleased with the results so far, and I am thankful for possibly adequate time to build up my immune system so as to eliminate all cancer cells, dysplasia, and atypia. Using Broffman's protocol and other supplemental and conjunctive approaches, I plan to be free of cancer five weeks from now when I have my TURBT.

In case you have forgotten the above quote is from Robert Heinlein's *Stranger in a Strange Land*, which is wonderful entertaining reading while you're recovering from any illness.

This morning I had another wonderful guided imagery session with Leslie Davenport. The focus of the session was on what guidance I need to make it through this period of waiting. Most of what came up was being in the present with my breathing ("breathing in, I'm healing myself, breathing out, I'm clear of cancer"). The other part of it seemed to come from my past experience with my son. My friend B. C. and I performed certain magical rituals that I think had an effect on his health. I'm now on the lookout for such magical thinking. At the group session which followed my guided imagery, this concept came out in a drawing I made of a healing spot in the Ozark Mountains in Arkansas. Perhaps tuning into that healing spot well enough will do the trick, but I certainly want to do some more exploring.

I came home to nap and then had a visit with A Ce Diamond. I plan to do a web page for his non-invasive form of Body Sculpture. Stay tuned!

### 3/30/97: Easter Sunday

I wasn't able to write anything yesterday because I was feeling quite badly. I felt like sleeping most of the day, which I did, even though D. and S. came from Arizona. They'll be here next weekend, though, and I will be better by then. I'm already better today, but the raw feeling inside my body persists. I still feel a lot like sleeping. Perhaps this is quite a normal response to 5FU and cisplatin. I haven't had too much nausea, and it has been quite controlled with Ativan.

About the best thing that I can recall about yesterday is that I was able to return to my belly breath quite frequently, in spite of feeling awful. I still remembered, "breathing in I'm healing myself, breathing out, I'm clear of cancer" or simply, "healing... clear", with each breath. This practice removes me from the remorse of having cancer and controls my discursive thinking quite a bit.

We had a pot luck at our house today. Our best friends showed up with the best food! I was still feeling like my insides were raw, so I tried to soothe my insides with Aloe Vera and Rescue Remedy. They worked a little, but not 100%. I was nervous about the Aloe Vera that was bought because of its potency and purity. I'm still wondering if T-Up is worth buying.

### 3/31/97: Off to Florida

My oldest daughter is off to Florida today with her best friend and her best friend's mother. My youngest has plans for the whole week. Just after she left, J. W., from my enneagram group was in Sausalito and stopped by to see me. We spent quite a long time together, reviewing each other's cancer treatments. She's reached to turning point in her cure and was very encouraging about my current status.

Unfortunately, the rawness inside my body continued to haunt me most of the day, but I tried to take a short walk and spend a few minutes in the sun with Itzzy. He was comforting and of great help when I needed to be taken to bed. We had a few quality moments of time together, as I could tell he was concerned.

Anna Halprin's class was again taught by her students. It was another great class, and my drawing was a "magic circle." I barely had enough energy to move, however.

### 4/1/97: My First Reiki!

To my surprise, Anne Pera, R. N., the massage therapist at Marin Radiation Oncology was a Reiki healer, as well. So I opted for a Reiki session which lasted about thirty-five minutes. I had planned to take a short walk after the healing, but I needed to lie down instead. The Reiki session seemed to realign my energy field, especially around my knees and bladder. Anne felt more inclined to work on my back side for she was able to feel the energy more cleanly.

My meditation has taken a slightly new twist today. It has transformed to, "Breathing in, I'm healing myself. Breathing out, I'm free of cancer," or "healthy... free!"

I was able to solve my bug this morning! Now I'm off on another one!

## 4/2/97: Gratitude

I spent most of the day today at NGC. The first person I saw when I arrived was my first boss and now Vice President of the whole Tools division, M. H. We spoke for about fifteen minutes, in which I explained my condition, and he congratulated me on the good bug fixing I had been doing. Then I felt motivated to express my gratitude for all the company has done for me since I became ill. I mentioned my boss and G. G., the chief technical officer. M. H. responded with such respect and grace that I was deeply moved. I am blessed to be working for such a forward looking company - one who takes pride in their employees, no matter what their physical condition.

I had lunch with my boss, and treated him for his kindness and generosity. I met with several other employees that I work with and by 3:00, I was so exhausted that I needed to leave. On the way home and on the way there, I listened to tapes by Thich Nhat Hanh.

At night, we went to a free preview of the movie, *The Saint*. It was fun, but a little much for one day yet.

## 4/3/97: Healing Support

Today I went to Cancerport again. The group was once again quite small, so just about everyone got a chance to speak. People asked how I was doing, and I had a long opportunity to explain what was going on with me. Basically, I told them that I had not recovered as quickly from the second chemotherapy and radiation as the first, but mentally and emotionally I was doing quite well. I still have difficult periods with my elimination and a lot of tiredness. I explained how my meditation and imagery work kept my mind focused in my body and away from morbid thoughts. I explained how radical cystectomy was the standard of treatment and that I had decided to take charge of my own case by doing the Shipley method and just how that worked. I told them how I used the web to find out information about my disease and as a means of tracking my healing progress.

Someone then asked me about how I felt about having cancer. I proceed to explain that my father had bladder cancer and died at the age of eighty-six from it, but that he had had a tumor in his bladder for perhaps twenty years. I told them about my son's metastatic Wilm's tumor, and that it was another form of urinary track cancer. Then I explained my sister's death due to Leukemia twenty-eight years ago and my mother's osteosarcoma. Finally, I mentioned that all my aunts and uncles died from cancer. Thus I felt that I had a genetic disposition towards getting cancer and that the stress brought about by the loss of my job 1993 probably brought it on.

The discussion turned more towards the alternative treatments that I am using and I spoke about specifically about Michael Broffman and Marty Rossman as partners in my care with the Marin Cancer Institute. I tried to explain that one did not have to believe in meditation or imagery for them to work, even though several people insisted that some level of belief was necessary. So I explained that just a people go to work out at the gym to keep their physical bodies in good shape, they could learn to quiet their mind with a little practice. Wonderfully enough, other people with imagery and/or meditation experience backed up my mini-lesson on meditation, and I felt safe enough to share the insight about "healthy cells grow all by themselves."

From there, I went to G. T. for another Functional Integration session. It was tremendously healing, once again, and Gail and I shared a lot with each other about our lives and our personal growth. I love working with her because she is so understanding and has such great hands. I bet she gives a hell of a massage!

Tonight I was supposed to meet my wife at M. C.'s house for dinner and a movie, but I really don't feel up to going out again. I think yesterday was too much for me and I still exhausted from the long drive to Menlo Park.

Well, "enough for today," as Bhagwan used to say!

### 4/4/97: Following the "*Yellow Stream!*"

Last night was quite difficult for me. I felt really exhausted and didn't like what was going on in my body. I prepared a modest meal and got in bed to read more of *That's Funny, You Don't Look Buddhist*. I enjoy it thoroughly, but the chapter on the holocaust moved me to tears and longing. I felt rejected by god and Jews as a child, but something is still trying to make itself felt in the way of devotional practice. I can't wait until my conversation with Sylvia Boorstein on April 15! One other thing about the book: If you take a combination of traits from my siblings, including myself, you get something that resembles the life of Sylvia and her family. David is orthodox and lives in St. Louis and is a grandpa. Joe is orthodox and lives in Israel with his family. Brenda is a drama therapist, and Manny is the owner of Art and Science of Computer Imaging - a very creative outlook!

My wife went with me to Leslie Davenport's cancer group. Many of the people in attendance were also at Cancerport the day before. During the meditation, I was filled with images of Hebrew school and the Miriam Hebrew Academy, which I hated so much. But I did remember and continue to reflect on one moment one fine day in April or May of 1946 or 1947 when I was filled with and experience of awe and wonder that has been with me all my life. I believe that this might have been my **first transcendental experience**, in which I became fully aware of the sun, the sky, the back yard of the academy, all of the other boys and girls playing their little games, the grass, and the brick garage with its attached brick ash pit. This moment was special for me, and I knew then that I was different from all the other boys and girls. I had no friends and played alone. At that point in my life I didn't know rejection, but I did feel left out. I used to sit in class and day dream about this and that, but never a clear image. I drew a picture of the garage and the ash pit and a boy playing ball.

In the afternoon, I went to a Feldenkrais session with Alan Sheets. Alan and I had worked together on an article which appeared in *Enneagram Monthly* on *The Enneagram of the Body*, which is Alan's method of teaching the enneagram. We had a really nice connection while we were working on the article and he expresses his gratitude for how much he appreciated my work.

Before the session, Alan asked me what I wanted to work on. I explained to him the importance of reality anchoring in the body, especially when you are ill, and that this is what I wanted to continue to work on. I told him about the weakness of my knees, lower back, and shoulders, and that this is what I wanted him to work on. For this session, Alan chose to work on my knees and lower back. I could feel the subtle movements as he proceeded to heal my body. The session was magnificent, but I really felt exhausted afterwards. One of the nicest moments came near the end when I could feel the energy flow from the bottoms of my feet where Alan was working all the way up to my skull. I believe that this has the wonderful effect of aiding lymphatic return and circulation.

Reality anchoring in the body is one of the foundations of the *Abhidhamma*, or Buddhist psychology. The principle is that out of all of our experience, what goes on in our bodies is of prime importance and it is what we share in common. It is based on the idea that we share reality from this common ground of being. We don't easily share thoughts, feeling, or emotions, but we all know what it is like to overeat, cut our fingers, burn our hands, or have a good night's sleep. Reality anchoring in the body provides us with a reality check on our condition. When we have a strong sense of reality anchoring in the body, we can proceed to manage our health care in a realistic way, without denial or fear.

## 4/5/97: I Love the Sounds of Spring

I woke up this morning and began my morning meditation, during which this poem came to me:
> *5:30 AM. The Sun rises across the Bay.*
> *The birds sing in the trees.*
> *I lie in my bed, breathing in, breathing out.*
> *I love the sounds of spring!*

I'm not much of a poet, but this one seems OK!

Today promises to be one with many visitors! D. and S. G. spent last night with us and planned to be with us most of the day. K. S. came with her two kids. We had a great lunch at Kitti's place, which seems to be our home away from home these days. Kitti was the chief chef at Comforts in San Anselmo. It seems that Comforts sold out about six months after Kitti opened his own place.

Later in the day, V. R. came with a friend of hers. V. is in my enneagram group and we have a deep affection for each other. She was so loving and compassionate that I hated to see her leave.

We went to A. and S. M.'s for dinner, but I really started to get exhausted after walking a lot of steps up into their house on Lombard Street.

## 4/6/97: A Mini Enneagram Lesson

My oldest daughter is returned from Miami today only three hours late! It's been six days since I've seen her, and by her silence I know that she is safe and having the time of her life.

I was supposed to have a massage this morning, but it got cancelled

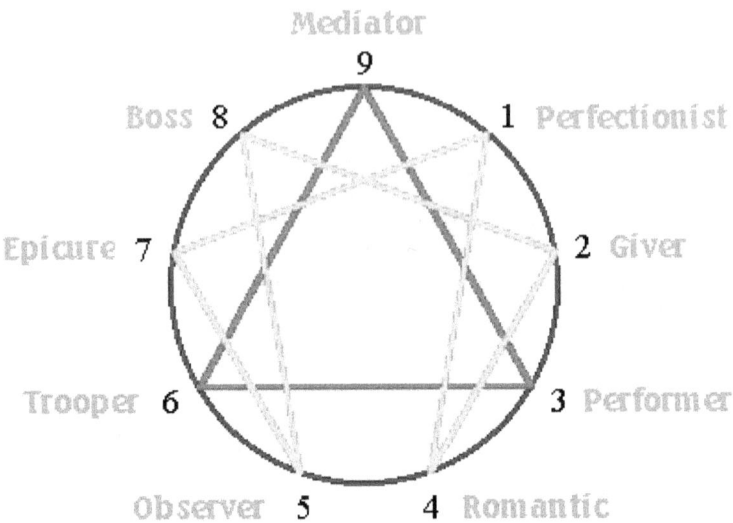

## The Enneagram of Personality Types

because of the birth of a new baby instead! Oh well! So instead, I thought I'd tell you what I've been thinking about lately according to the enneagram.

The enneagram is a diagram that describes nine personality types shown in the diagram to the left. Each personality type has associated with it a vice and a virtue. In my case, since I'm a *trooper*, my vice is *fear* and my virtue is *courage*! This whole cancer issue for me has been a question of courage to face and accept my condition and find the necessary faith to take charge of my own treatment plan. By learning your enneagram point, you can discover what your vices and virtues are, and manage your case with the appropriate actions for your personality type. For more information, please see my enneagram pages.

I received another email from R. M., a 59 year old man in New Zealand who has bladder cancer and doesn't want radical cystectomy either. We have been corresponding for more than a month, and the message I received today was quite special. He shared with me that he too had been a follower of Rajneesh, and offered many of Bhagwan's meditations to me. I wrote back that I was called Swami Deva Ninad by Rajneesh in 1975 and knew all about the meditations. I'm waiting to hear back from him!

## 4/7/97: Seeds of Enlightenment

This morning, I managed to get in about forty-five minutes of tennis! It was difficult to manage my energy, but I'm feeling stronger every day.

By the time I went to Anna Halprin's class, however, my gut was churning and my energy was quite low. Fortunately, we spent a lot of time during check-in because there were several new people there, including J. B., the mother of my daughter's best friend.

The movement segment began with sitting in or chairs and doing deep breathing exercises. I gradually picked up to where we were supporting our faces with our hands and keeping our hands in touch with our bodies. At a certain point, I felt the desire to do a modified form Zen prostrations as an expression of gratitude. I continued moving about on the floor for quite a while, returning to the prostrated position quite frequently. Then the movement picked up all over the room and my energy began to accelerate. Mostly, I was dancing alone, but there were quite wonderful encounters with other dancers, and soon, most of the group was dancing together. I spontaneously moved into the third stage of the "chaotic meditation" that I learned at the Ashram from Rajneesh. This is the stage where "With raised arms, jump up and down shouting the mantra HOO!...HOO!...HOO! as deeply as possible, coming from the bottom of your belly." Most of the people joined my in this movement, and I was filled with images of the Ashram and Bhagwan.

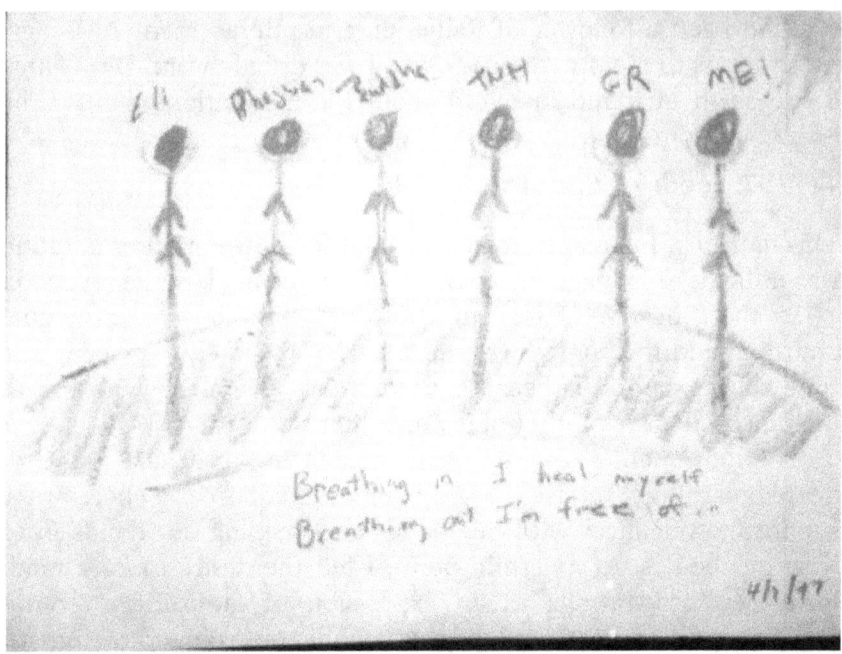

After the movement segment settled down with a group circle, we did our drawings. I wanted to draw a group of people dancing together at the Ashram in Pune, but I knew that I lacked the artistic talents to make it happen, so I just started drawing orange faces, which transformed into six vibrant flowers with roots in the earth and healthy leaves on the stalks - all reminding me of "healthy cells growing all by themselves." On top of each flower, I wrote the name of one of my major teachers along my path.

The first flower was dedicated to Father Eli, from whom I learned the trance work that forms the foundation for guided imagery well enough to teach it to over two hundred people since 1973. He told me that he had taught both Jose Silva of Silva Mind Control, which I had learned in 1971, and L. Ron Hubbard, founder of Scientology, which I studied between 1968 and 1971.

The second flower was dedicated to Bhagwan Shree Rajneesh, also known as Osho. I spent the summer of 1975 in Poona and was given the name, Swami Deva Ninad. I have collected more than four hundred tapes and twenty-five books of his lectures.

The third and fourth flowers were dedicated to the Buddha and Thich Nhat Hanh, respectively. Since 1985, I have been devoted to

Buddhism in general and Zen and Vipassana meditation in particular. I love the way Thay has interpreted the sutra on *Mindfulness of Breathing*. My own meditation is totally inspired by him.

The fifth flower was dedicated to Gabrielle Roth, a former student of Anna Halprin, and an internationally known shaman. I studied with her in 1975 - 1976, as we shared a common interest in Bhagwan and the enneagram. I was scheduled to assist her at a workshop at Eselan in June of 1996, but on that very day, my son went into the hospital for his Wilm's tumor surgery. What a shock it was for me to have to change my plans and spend the time in the hospital instead. Gabrielle harnessed the energy of her workshop at Eselan and all of her remaining workshops that year to perform healing circles for my son. I have been devoted to her since then and have felt a great sense of gratitude.

The last flower, I dedicated to myself, as I am now my own guru. I am learning a lot every day from my illness and my efforts to keep my mind focused on healing. Naturally, I look to the other teachers for inspiration, but most things are coming from deep inside me.

As a result of the drawing, my meditation has changed slightly, once again. It now goes, "Breathing in I heal, breathing out I'm free," or simply, "healthy... free."

## 4/8/97: Two-Pointedness!

Today I went in for a check-up with Dr. Gullion, and saw Dr. Bobbie Head instead. My blood counts were good and there is no need to worry about infection. I asked about a more complete exam, but I was told that this was only to check the blood counts.

I had a second massage at the Cancer Institute with Anne Pera. This time she did a "Metamorphosis" on my feet, hands, skull and back. She has such a light healing touch that I can recommend her highly. She's really present when she works on you and you can feel the healing energy in her hands.

My session with Leslie Davenport turned out to be quite magnificent! I spent about one half hour simply describing the state of my healing. I told her about the work with Anna Halprin, the Feldenkrais work, my contact with R. M. in New Zealand, and my "seeds of enlightenment," which seemed to thrill her quite a bit. I talked about *That's Funny, You Don't Look Buddhist*, and some feelings about my family of origin and childhood experiences. I expressed how I felt rejected as a child by my family, school mates, the kids at Hebrew school and Sunday school, and by God. I explored these feelings without regret, but with a sense of longing. These feelings were overwhelmed by my new sense of love for myself and the work I am doing to heal.

In the guided imagery portion, Leslie began with these inspiring words:

> *"As we begin, just notice where you are as we start... where your attention seems to be clustered... And to engage with the knowledge that you have the freedom and the power to focus your awareness... And feel how each breath, each moment has never been lived before, has never been breathed before... acknowledging the newness... the presence of each part of the breath... each moment of the breath... And to begin to also sense that balance between your focusing of attention and the receptivity... the active, the receptive, of any guidance that may come through at any point... And staying a little longer with the breath and feel how the in breath carries strength into your body, clarity into you mind, stability into your emotions... connectedness to that deep sense of yourself... And how the out breath by its very nature has that cleansing, clearing, letting go qualities... And allowing yourself to begin to tune into your body with the fresh eyes and the fresh sensing that arise out of this moment... And to go ahead and allow your focus to go right into the place in your body most in need of healing... And just to allow images to form which may be familiar or new..."*

I tuned into my bladder and had the same images as when I felt "healthy cells growing all by themselves." Then I noticed a white spot in the area where the tumor was and decided to focus all of my attention on that area. My attention became so one-pointed that I began to feel waves of bliss, which I again used to support the growth of healthy cells. When I expressed how I was doing, Leslie said, "Well, it's actually two-pointed because I'm putting mine there too!"

### 4/9/97: Every Day I Get Better and Better!

Today is the first day I didn't feel the need to nap. This is possibly because I took a walk by the Bay in Sausalito. I found my favorite spot to sit for fifteen minutes doing my "healing... free" meditation. It was very pleasant and the time went by very fast. There were times while I was meditating that I felt tired, but they passed, just like all my passing thoughts. The experience of impermanence was brought home again by the changing thoughts and feelings of being tired. I then did the strengthening exercises at the same location as my sitting meditation, and felt quite strong.

## 8 - ALMOST NORMAL LIFE

### 4/10/97: Feel Good to Heal Good!

I woke up very early this morning, feeling almost normal! Before I had cancer, I would wake up early, go down into my office, and begin working. This morning, I followed the same procedure, in spite of having taken a sleeping pill last night. Aside from Cancerport, later this morning, I have an Evolutionary Circle meeting tonight, for the first time in about a month.

Cancerport was a very moving experience for me, as mothers spoke of children they wanted to see graduate and get married! This is also my experience, as one daughter graduates middle school in June and the other next June. I want to be there when they have grandchildren! I felt that it was appropriate to share my guided imagery session about "healthy cells growing all by themselves" again, and once more, it was received with great interest and care.

Several of us went to eat together at Taqueria San Jose in San Rafael. If you have never been there, you're in for a treat. This is a real, down-home taco place that serves fresh orange juice and fresh carrot juice made to order. I also enjoy their soft tacos more than anywhere else.

During the discussion, I heard about one woman who is surviving cervical cancer for over twenty-two years, with eleven recurrences! One of the women I had lunch with has survived over eleven years with hers!

At the Evolutionary Circle, I showed a ten minute segment from *In Search of ... Faith Healing* from 1980, in which my son's Wilm's tumor was the subject of research. The group was moved by his amazing healing and felt very inspired. I next spoke for a long time about my healing process, including "healthy cells grow all by themselves," and other anecdotes. The love and support I felt transformed my feeling of exhaustion into as state of excitement. We all shared where were mentally and emotionally and left with good feelings for each other.

A friend of R. W.'s was there who is a Reiki healer and does laying on of the hands healing. I look forward to next week's meeting where she will teach us some of her healing techniques.

This group has been going now for almost two years! In we try to support the goals and desires of each of the members with our thoughts and imagery. Next week we should have T. W. and her husband also.

## 4/11/97: It's Only Tennis!!

I'm going to miss Leslie's group this morning to play tennis! I played for almost two hours and I can still do my work for the day! It's so nice to do something you enjoy so much!

## 4/12/97: When the Iron Bird Flies...

Last night, our neighbors visited us. J. G. told me that she was invited to a dinner with the Dalai Lama sometime in June! She said that she would try to get me invited without having to pay the $500 per plate. I was thrilled at the prospect.

I spent the morning working and playing tennis with the guys at Eastwood Park. It was wonderful again! I felt welcome and played quite well under the circumstances.

During my afternoon meditation, it dawned on me that both Thich Nhat Hanh and the Dalai Lama are exiles, from Viet Nam and Tibet, respectively. This reminded me of what Padmasambhava said in the eighth century,

*"When the iron bird flies and horses run on wheels, the Tibetan people will be scattered like ants across the world and the Dharma will come to the land of the Red Man!"*

Alfred Toynbee has said that the most significant thing to happen in the 20th century is the coming of Buddhism to the West.

Tonight, we are going out for a special dinner and a concert with the Ying Quartet.

## 4/13/97: Reframing a Bad Day

I'm having a bad cancer day today. I woke up feeling tense and anxious and it took me around two hours to get in touch with what the problem was. I was feeling all of the financial pressure of paying for my cancer care and at the same time, keeping my household in order. Before I had cancer, we were already stretched to the limit, having chosen to spend our money on our childrens' education. Now, with the added stress of medical bills not covered by insurance, I'm really feeling the pinch. Just talking with friends and family and writing about it relieves the pain a little, and now I'm feeling more centered.

I got another email from R. M. in New Zealand. He had his TUR and it went well.

I managed to get myself out to play a little tennis this afternoon. This, combined with the advice from M. C., who gave me the massages when I returned home from the hospital on January 31, helped to finally lift me out of the bad day. M. C. suggested that I reframe my financial worries into gratitude that the cancer was found in time and pay the bills with thanksgiving for the opportunity to explore my life and bring my cancer under control. I took her suggestions to heart and now I'm feeling much better.

I also spoke with my brother, Manny. He gave me some valuable suggestions for copyrighting this work and finding a publisher! I'm really grateful for his suggestions.

### 4/14/97: The Frog on the Leaf...

Compared to yesterday, this was a fine day, but I was still haunted by the cost of cancer. I worked in the morning and then went to have a session with Alan Sheets. He worked on my knees, lower back, shoulders, cranium, and bladder. The session was very relaxing and I didn't feel the need to nap for the rest of the day.

From Alan's office, I met G. S. at the California Conservatory of Music to pick up twenty copies of *Yellow Stream* which my son had made for me. These copies go through the beginning of chapter eight, and are expressly for the purpose of finding a publisher for the web site as a book. I might change the title to "*Healthy Cells Grow All By Themselves*" before final publication.

From there, I went to Golden Gate Park for a walk and a time to be alone in nature. I just had a feeling that this would be better for me than rushing back home to get more work done on the Sniffer. On the way to the Redwood Grove, I passed a small pond with beautiful, broad leaves in it. Perhaps they were water lilies not yet in bloom. It was a beautiful pond, and then I noticed a frog sitting on one of the leaves. The frog was as big as the leaf, about three inches long, and two and one-half inches wide. I stood and watched the frog for several minutes. When I thought about it later, I thought about this poem:

> *The frog on a leaf*
> *In the pond*
> *In the Arboretum*
> *Just sitting*

*Doing Zazen*

I wandered off to the Redwood Grove and found a place to sit on the stump of a redwood tree to meditate. I was surrounded by redwood trees and sat next to another pond (no frog) for about fifteen minutes. Then I searched out the incense cedar tree that my son and I often visited when he was young. In fact, it was after playing in that tree that he told me something was wrong with his stomach, and a few weeks later he was diagnosed with Wilm's Tumor. I hugged the tree and offered prostrations to it for helping heal my son and now I was asking for its help to heal me. The prostration was humbling and healing at the same time. Hopefully, no one saw me doing such a strange thing.

Next I visited the moon viewing platform which juts out over another pond (no frogs here either) in hopes of running into Itzzy, who often does *Tai Chi* on that platform. Then it was time to go and I slowly left the Arboretum being mindful of each step and each breath.

At night, I went to Anna Halprin's class and offered her the first printed copy of *Yellow Stream*. She seemed really grateful. The class got off to a slow start, with Anna's boom box not working. We sat and did breathing exercises and I noticed that several people were having a tough time. I thought that this would have been a good evening for a long check-in, but we moved forward anyway. Anna spent much of her time with the woman that was having the most difficulty, and I enjoyed dancing to the rhythms of the drums that were playing when we finally had some music.

My drawing came right out of my gut. I looked at the box of crayons and noticed that there was a small piece of a thick, red crayon that appealed to me. I picked it up and started drawing bold, thick curved lines that eventually resembled a large hourglass, but in reality, it was my anger of the cost of cancer coming through. I wrote, "I want to see my anger red!" I wanted to have an intuitive feeling for why I was so pissed off about the cost of treatment, or at least have someone tell me what I was feeling. The expressing of anger in the drawing was quite strong, and I received a lot of good feedback about it during the ensuing discussion.

As people shared their drawings, I felt the group coming closer together. I stated, "I finally feel that the group is coming together. Even though we are still having a tough time, we are having a tough time together." Many agreed with my statement.

I headed home feeling much better and with a strong desire to write.

However, as I walked in the door the phone rang and the call was from New York. I was told about a healer named Winefred Wager, who I'm supposed to call tomorrow to see if she can help me "long distance!" I also had a message from Dean Ornish, but I haven't spoken with him yet. He is starting a prostate cancer study with Dr. Carroll.

## 4/15/97: Who Are the People in Your Neighborhood?

My wife and I met Sylvia Boorstein at the Good Earth at 9:00 in the morning. We had such a delightful time speaking with her about everything from dharma to family drama. She is obviously a wonderful and caring person who is enjoying a happy life between Buddhism and Judaism. We talked about our favorite prayers in the synagogue and it turns out that the service for replacing the torah is both of our favorites. It talks about the torah being, "a tree of life and everyone that upholds it is happy!"

I spoke to her about my practice and she thought that it was wonderful to have "healing... free" as a meta-program throughout my breathing. I wanted to speak more to her about my practice, but the time seemed to fly by. At one point, she said, "We must learn to cultivate boundless love rather than just adhere to a structure." We were talking about the practices of the orthodox that seem to follow the structure more than their hearts. Later, she said, "It's not in the liturgy, it's in the heart!" She told me about Elat Chayyim in upstate New York, which is supposed to be like a Jewish Eselan. It's funny, but I don't have any desire to go there. I'm sure I'll see her again quite soon.

My massage was cancelled, so I worked in Leslie Davenport's office until our appointment at 1:00. We worked on the financial issues in my life, which was very appropriate for what had been happening over the weekend. I had images of my grandfather on my mother's side, who seemed to be the most generous person in the family. After all, he was in his eighties and well taken care of by my mother and my uncle, Sam Sandmel, the Reformed Rabbi and publisher of many books on Jews and Jesus. But my money problems seem to go deeper into my childhood and relate to matters about feeling unworthy and rejected. There is still a lot of work to do about this area, and I plan to continue until it is resolved. One thing that Leslie said at the end of the session was that I should really focus on things that I can change in my life and let go of things that I have no control over. I thought this was appropriate advice at the time, and I've heard it many times before.

The most significant thing that happened in the session was just before the end. I could feel the waves of sadness starting to overcome me, even though I was still focused on my breathing, doing, "healing... free". The feelings came, got very intense, and then started to melt away, all under the eyes of mindfulness. I experienced the impermanence of the rise and fall of the sad feelings in a way that had never touched me so deeply before. This is, according to my understanding, the text book practice of *vipassana* meditation.

My session with G. T. was wonderful once again. We worked on my back and pelvis, and I could feel the energy shifting, as she would go through the various steps of the lesson. We are developing a wonderful connection of mutual love and support as we continue to work together. Since she's so fond of dance and art, I invited her to Anna's class on April 28 to come as one of my support persons.

I came home thoroughly and totally exhausted, so I headed straight for a "mind story." This time I settled into my breathing and was able put my worries out of my mind to get a clear picture of my bladder's "healthy cells growing all by themselves!" I felt rested and much, much better at the end of the "mind story!"

At night, we went to a dinner party at S. and C.'s just two houses away. Ten of our best neighbors were gathered together for a very nice time.

## 4/16/97: Hi Ho, Hi Ho, It's Off to Work I Go

R. T., my boss, and I are met to discuss my raise and bonus, so I went to Menlo Park for the day. Marty Rossman was traveling to some Alternative Medicine conference in Orlando, so I drove him to the airport, which is on my way. This gave me a chance to chat with Marty about my life and ask him about his. The main point of our discussion was the effectiveness of guided imagery in my cure. Of course, he's the master! When I asked him about Yellow Stream, he said that he was very impressed with the resources section.

I met my son for lunch at the Uptime Cafe at NGC. I had lunch cards from when I taught a class at NGC, so we got to pig out on cafeteria food! He was fairly talkative about his life, but we didn't discuss my illness at length. He is going to sing for G. T.'s mother on Friday night.

So, the day turned out to be kind of a normal workday, as my life is becoming more and more normal and my symptoms are affecting my daily activities less and less. For example, I didn't have time for a mind story today, but I compensated by going to bed by 8:30.

### 4/17/97: The Ups and Downs of Cancer

This morning, I had the most wonderful massage from Elyse. This was the third in a series given to me by M. C. when she first heard about my cancer. The massage was sterling! Elyse did some amazing work on my back and abdomen. I feel that she may be one of the best around.

I had a different kind of session with Leslie Davenport today. She used EMDR (Eye Movement Desensitization and Reprocessing) as a therapeutic tool. The technique involves random eye movements induced by the therapist while the patient is focusing on a troublesome emotional or physical problem. The goal is to desensitize the brain to the feelings associated with the event in order to allow the brain to reprocess the event in present time.

As for my session, I was dealing with five issues that came to light while I was reading *Getting Well Again*. The issues related to stress around losing a job in 1993 and changing from consulting to a full-time position. In addition, I have been undergoing therapy since then to recover my sense of personal power and have therefore come in to quite a conflict with my spouse, who always wants to be in control. The other two major stresses in my life have been in the area of financial worries and interpersonal relationships. During the therapy, I was aware of how all of these issues were interconnected, and that the missing ingredient was "unconditional love." Leslie offered that she had found this through her spiritual practices and that I possibly could do the same. I left feeling a little depressed, but now that I've had a nap and a chance to write about my experience, I feel a lot better.

Later in the evening, I went to a meeting of my Evolutionary Circle. The meeting focused on healing, especially laying on of the hands, and other methods. We just had time to heal two members, neither of which was I, but I got a lot out of tuning into the other members and finding a way to offer my healing energy. I felt that B. M. needed energy around her thymus, and so I moved my hand in a healing motion around her thymus and then placed the ammonite fossil that Barbara Rose Billings gave me over her thymus. Then I touched and tapped her sternum. At the end of the healing, she shared that she thought that something was indeed going on with her immune system.

## 4/18/97: All Things are Impermanent!

Today was rather a strange day. I was supposed to play tennis at 8:30 A. M., but the ground was wet, so we postponed it to 10:00 A. M. By 10:00, the courts had not dried, so tennis was cancelled. By now, I was going over some bugs with a colleague at work, and by the time we finished our conversation, it was too late to go to Leslie's group. So I settled into work until about 1:45, when my wife called to tell me she was having car trouble and I needed to pick up the girls. So, off to the tennis courts I went for just about an hour! At last!

I didn't take time to relax this afternoon. I got caught up in computer stuff and now it's dinnertime! I guess I won't make Anna Halprin's open house this evening.

## 4/19/97: Birthday Greetings

Today was my wife's birthday and S. G.'s Bat Mitzvah. The Bat Mitzvah was a joyous occasion and many people wished me well. They were happy that I appeared to look so well and continue to visualize my complete recovery.

When I got home, I felt quite exhausted. I proceeded to do a "mind story" using Leslie Davenport's tape. Not too much else is happening on the healing front today!

## 4/20/97: Overprotection

When I was a boy of around twelve or thirteen, I studied and played the game of chess. I studied the masters like Lasker, Reinfeld, Alekhine, Botvinnik and Capablanca. In fact, when Reshevsky played a simultaneous exhibition at Purdue University in 1959, I played him to a tie by playing the Lasker variation of the Queen's Gambit Declined. My favorite master was Aaron Nimzovich, who published My System in 1925. This was my favorite book on the subject and I studied it long and hard. One of the strategies that Nimzovich taught was called overprotection. He maintained that if you have a pawn in a strong position, especially in the center of the board, you should do everything in your power to overprotect that pawn, which, in turn would lead to a very strong position. Overprotection became my primary strategy in chess, and perhaps in life.

Overprotection is a good strategy for raising children if you consider expressing your love and affection for them consistently throughout their childhood. I'm not talking about protecting them from the outside world so much as assuring them that they are loved and cared for in a way in which they feel secure and protected. My girls and boy have been raised this way and are wonderful people.

I think that overprotection is a good strategy for healing from cancer also. What I mean here is that the more you can do for yourself, the better. For me, this means being a support group junkie, doing "mind stories," having guided imagery sessions, doing Feldenkrais and other massage therapies, acupuncture, and all of the other activities I'm engaged in to support and overprotect my health.

I came to this realization early this morning after a very difficult night of little sleep. I was looking deeply into my feelings and remembered how I played chess and bridge as a youngster.

I studied the game so much so that I could feel like a winner. I had felt like such a looser as a child that I needed something to win at and I chose chess. Almost every time I played a good game with a good player with a chance to win, I would get heart palpitations and start to shake. I would get very nervous and feel compelled to win. I needed to win at something. This attitude and nervousness carried over into my college days at Purdue University to the game of bridge. I quickly became one of the best bridge players on campus, but winning was still an issue. When Mike Sears and I entered a tournament in Terra Haute, Indiana, I was nervous and shaking as usual, and we did not win. Mike was very disappointed in me. However, when Charles Goren visited Purdue, I was his partner in a tournament and we won.

Now my life is on the line and I'm playing for keeps. I get the same heart palpitations and shaking when I think of the possibility of actually helping someone with my ideas and guidance. I get nervous when I think about publishing this web site as a book and actually speaking to people about how they can learn to make appropriate decisions for their medical treatment. Now that the word is out, I may be able to control my nervousness and shaking enough to heal myself and realize my goal to deliver this message far and wide. This is serious stuff, and I am committed to getting well again. My girls are still young enough that they need overprotection - overprotection in the sense of feeling loved and protected.

### 4/21/97: The First Night of Passover

I was able to play three sets of tennis this morning, but I was so exhausted that it took me more than two hours to recover. I took a long bath and the got into bed for a long "mind story." Both of these were very relaxing and I found myself quite able to concentrate on my breathing and visualizing healing in my bladder. My poem became:
> Lying still,
> Breathing in, Breathing out,
> Healthy cells grow all by themselves.
> I am free of cancer.

The meditation became "healthy cells grow all by themselves" on the in breath and "I'm free of cancer" on the out breath, or simply, "healthy... free."

In the evening, we went over to A. and S. M.'s house for a lovely sader. I was able to participate fully, and even had a few cups of wine. It was a very enjoyable evening.

I'm still having sleep problems, however.

### 4/22/97: Weird Old Women Who Wear Purple!

Today I went to Leslie Davenport to work on my sleep problem. She led me in a hypnotherapy session which focused on deep relaxation and then led me into several visualizations that seemed to help me recover my ability to let go and allow myself to sleep. The tape recording was messed up, however, so I am going to have to reconstruct the session from memory while it is still fresh.

From focusing on deeply relaxing my physical body she went into deeply relaxing my mind through a technique of unraveling a loosely woven fabric of burlap or some similar substance. The purpose of this was to unravel the mind from its objects of attention. Next, we went deeper with a countdown followed by a visualization of a relaxing place. I chose China Beach in Point Lobos State Reserve.

The final scene was a library in my mind in which there were books of a positive nature on the right side of me and books of not such a positive nature on the left. The books on the left were stories about stress, illness, heartaches, pain, suffering, and the like. I took each of these books one by one and placed them in a receptacle which was then taken out of the library for good!

I came out of the session feeling very relaxed and as if I had taken a nap. I'm sure there was more to the session, so I'm going to ask Leslie about it and try to recover the tape.

Later, I went to see G. T.. She did a Feldenkrais session on twisting of my spine, which was very good. She also showed me exercises for my back and knees. While we were working together, she spoke about how much Feldenkrais has helped stroke victims. During the discussion, she mentioned that she thought she'd be around to be a weird old lady dressed in purple! I love doing work with Gail, but I won't see her until May 15 because she'll be in Feldenkrais training.

In the evening, my wife and I went to separate support groups at the Center for Attitudinal Healing in Sausalito. The support group I attended was the "Life Threatened" and my wife attended the "Care Givers" group. I first contacted The Center for Attitudinal when my son had Wilm's tumor back in 1976 and spoke with the founder, Dr. Jerry Jampolsky. Later, 1987 or 1988, my wife and I completed the Volunteer Training, but we got busy with our young children and never did much with the Center.

The support group was different from the others I've been attending in that it started and ended with everyone holding hands and one of the facilitators offering a message of hope. I enjoyed that aspect. When I had an opportunity to share, I really felt supported. Everyone was interested in my meditation of "healthy... free" and invited me to teach it, but as time was limited, I'll have to wait until another opportunity presents itself. I think people felt inspired by my story.

## 4/23/97: To Click or Not to Click...

Today was a very nice day! I went to Menlo Park around 11:00 A. M. and spoke with my boss once more about my annual review. Next, my son came for lunch and we had a nice time with the V. P. of my group. I received such tremendous support from everyone at work today that it really made me feel happy.

My little enneagram support group met in the afternoon. This was the first time we were all together for a very long time, and it really felt wonderful. In this group, we use our combined knowledge of the enneagram to help each other through good times and times that are not so good. We were all trained by Helen Palmer and completed our certification in 1991. We have been meeting regularly since September of 1994.

V. R. was describing how she had used email to end one relationship and begin another. At each step of the way, she had to decide on whether or not to send a specific message to one of her friends. This gave rise to the phrase of the day, "to click or not to click!" (Another example of "to click or not to click" occurred in the morning. I had just pressed the send button on an email message to D. K. when he phoned me to answer the question I was asking in the email!) As I shared what was going on with me, I felt totally supported, and each of us got enough time to share what we wanted to.

### 4/24/97: The Mother Ship

Last night, I had a dream. In the dream I was running away from an impending nuclear disaster to a space ship that was to take a number of people to safety. The "mother ship" had a lift that would allow one person at a time to be speedily transported into the ship. I noticed that the entry mechanism was rather weak and decided to redesign it. As I did so, the space ship seemed to grow in diameter and I was able to try out my new designs rather easily. Naturally, I woke before the disaster. I wonder what it all means.

At Cancerport today, I offered a copy of *Yellow Stream* to the group. I explained how each day had its own title and that some of them were quite funny. I shared how the book became known as *Yellow Stream* and everyone laughed. Earlier, someone mentioned that laughter was really good for healing, so we had plenty of it!

At night, we had another meeting of our Evolutionary Circle. The theme was once again based on healing through laying on of the hands. Before we actually did any healing work, we each had an opportunity to check in with the group. I could feel such love and support from everyone, as I shared what had happened in the last week. We are such an unlikely group of people that somehow we've managed to stay together for over a year now.

### 4/25/97: Bubbles of Energy

Leslie Davenport's group today was quite special. She led a guided imagery experience which was quite similar to the one I had earlier this week. We started with deep breathing, as usual, and switched to relaxing the body, starting with the eyes, working up to the forehead and to the top of the head. Then we moved to our face and then on down to the feet and toes. From there, she had us imagine bubbles of energy rising from our fully relaxed feet and legs on up through our torso and winding up at the top of our heads. The visualization was very effective for me, and I felt very relaxed during the whole process. I probably could have fallen asleep several times. I later found out that most of the people in the room felt a deep sense of relaxation also.

In response to a question from one of the members of the group, I had an opportunity to speak about managing your own health care and how to make appropriate medical decisions. I explained how I had to make a tough decision back in early February regarding radical cystectomy versus the Shipley approach with I eventually decided upon. I also spoke about integrative medicine as the approach I took. This gave rise to comments by many other people supporting what I had to say and enhancing my viewpoint. I shared that I really wanted to come to the group mostly when I was feeling good so I could share my healing experiences with other people and not be so needy. All in all, I felt really supported and that I had contributed to the healing experience of others in the room.

### 4/26/97: A Family Gathering

I played tennis this morning in Eastwood Park with the gang that was there. I was really in the "zone" today! I made a lot of shots simply by not thinking too much about them, which is exactly the space I like to be in when I play tennis. Again, it took me two hours to recover. I took an hour bath and also slept for about an hour.

In the evening, we went to my brother's house in Los Altos for a little sader. My son and his girlfriend were there, along with my sister, her husband, my brother's daughter with her entire family, and my brother's girl friend with her son. The gathering was very nice and quite spiritual. Somehow, it felt good for us all to be together to celebrate the festival of freedom.

### 4/27/97: Call from an Old Friend

This morning, I received a call from an old friend, Rabbi Zalman Schachter, who is now on the faculty at the Narpoa Institute. He called me because of an email that he received from Sylvia Boorstein. Zalman was quick to wish me well in my recovery, and his demeanor was full of loving-kindness. I really appreciated hearing from him at this time.

Later in the day, I helped my daughter with her school project on "Zen Buddhism - It's Beliefs and Effect on Society." I really enjoyed reading the material with her and helping her understand the concepts of Buddhism, in general, and Zen Buddhism in particular. The quote which really got to me this time through was,

*"This earth on which we stand, is the promised Lotus land,*
*And this very body is the body of the Buddha.*

Bhagwan spoke quite often on this subject, and I feel connected to the spirit of the quote.

Tomorrow starts another chapter!

## 9 - THE BIG QUESTION

### 4/28/97: Don Alejandro

This week and next week will determine the future course of my treatment. The Shipley protocol calls for another TUR around May 6, to determine if there is any cancer in my bladder. The question for Dr. Neuwirth is, "Is my bladder free of cancer?" If the answer is "yes", then I am to proceed with more chemotherapy and radiation. This phase is known as "consolidation CFI," where CFI stands for cisplatin, 5FU, and irradiation. If the answer is not "yes", then Dr. Neuwirth will probably recommend "radical cystectomy," which I want to avoid.

To help me cope with such a decision, I went to see a Peruvian shaman by the name of Don Alejandro this morning. The session took place in Sebastopol, about 50 miles north of Sausalito. I had in interpreter who translated Don Alejandro's Spanish into English for me on the fly - as he was speaking. This was a little confusing at first, but I eventually got used to it. I asked him the questions on the list in Appendix 4. [**NOTE**: The questions for this appendix can be found on the *Mindulfness In Healing* website at http://mindfulnessinhealing.org/appendix-4.]

In the session, Don Alejandro told me that my disease was hereditary. Then I explained to him how my sister died of Leukemia, my mother of an osteosarcoma, my dad of bladder cancer, and how my son survived kidney cancer. Don Alejandro recommended that I continue with the chemotherapy and radiation, if that was required. He felt for sure that I would be cured of cancer, but that it may be a slow process. He said that there would probably be more than one looking into my bladder for cancer. He gave me advice on what to eat: no cold drinks, no red meat, fish in small quantities, and no seafood (my favorite). I should eat steamed or raw vegetables to make up the calories that I need to take in. Cold drinks cause the digestive system to clam up and can cause inflammation in the bladder. I don't quite understand this, but maybe Michael Broffman can explain it to me. He suggested I take cat's claw, which I already knew about. I'll also check this out with Michael Broffman.

He said that I should maintain peace of mind and let all of my problems go. He asked me if I followed any religion, and I naturally told him that I followed Buddhism. He didn't make a comment about this, but I'm sure it figured into the psychic equation.

Prior to doing his psychic healing, Don Alejandro had me drink an herbal beverage that was quite bitter. I was expecting apple juice! Then I lay down on the bed and he proceeded to heal me according to his methods. He first explored my bladder area with his hands and then began a chant in a strange language that could have been mistaken for Hebrew. The chant lasted about five minutes and was very soothing. I noticed that he was sitting with his hands in the prayer position while chanting.

The next thing I knew was that he was laying his hands on my bladder area. After a while, I got the idea to open psychically to him, and I felt him penetrate my defenses. I found myself smiling during the process, and furthermore, I maintained a focus on my breathing with "healthy... free..." Some of his manipulations of my bladder area began to hurt, and I tightened up a bit. Then I realized that this was part of the healing process and I relaxed into it. His work proceeded without further hindrance from me, and soon it was over. He pronounced the healing complete, and, at the same time, ended the session.

I left Sebastopol almost immediately, as I felt that I needed time to integrate what he said and what he did. We came straight home and I did a "mind story" about the healing. My feeling now is that he did major good and I would definitely see him again. By the way, the tape recorder was on "pause," so I didn't get any of the conversation. However, the essence of the treatment was the healing, not the words.

In a way, I am now better prepared for a bad answer from Dr. Neuwirth, because Don Alejandro had said that I may have to have my bladder looked into more than once. I'm not sure if he was seeing the follow-up cystoscopy exams, or another TURBT.

In the afternoon, I went to see Dr. Neuwirth, who was quite pleased with how I looked. However, he did not examine me and his scheduler made a point of my having a physical exam with Dr. Belknap before the surgery next week on May 8. He did say that he was willing to have Julie Motz in the operating room with him. He even mentioned that she was in the operating room with a friend of his last week.

For those of you who haven't heard of Julie Motz, I'll give you a little run down of what I know from reading the *Pacific Sun* article from April 23, to April 29, 1997. The article basically states that Julie enters the operating room with the surgeon and does laying on of the hands healing during the surgery. She is the first to use energy healing in the operating room. She works primarily with cancer and heart disease patients. She is giving a lecture at Marin General Hospital on May 8 at 7:00 P. M. I'm trying to use my connection with Leslie Davenport to get to speak with Julie Motz about visiting me during my surgery next week.

Julie Motz called me a little later and said that she would love to work with me, but she can't do it on May 8. I'm now trying to reschedule my surgery for May 9 to have her there and participate in my healing experience. Maybe I can even get her to write a preface to *Yellow Stream*!

In the evening, I attended Anna Halprin's class. As Anna was receiving an award from her peers, the class was taught by Jordy. She taught a class before, and this one

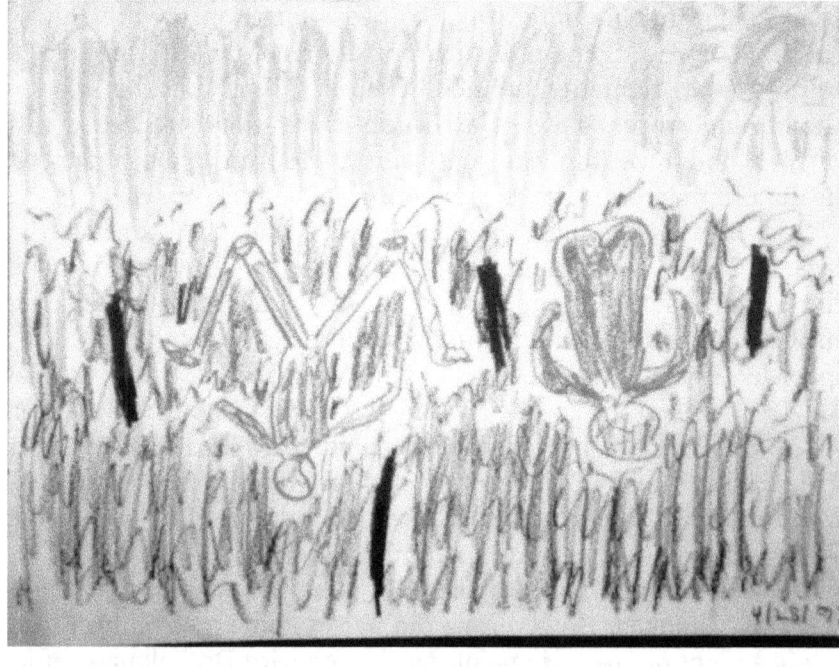

was quite good. The theme of the evening was getting in touch with parts of our bodies that were free and not so free. I identified my knees as being not so free and my buttocks as free. We expressed these parts through writing, movement, working in pairs, and drawing. I drew this picture. Then go to http://www.mindfulnessinhealing.org/wp-content/uploads/AH970428r.jpg to get a rotated version. Quite by accident, the picture works from both orientations. In the first, we see two people lying in the grass with a blue sky above them. In the second, the people are still lying in the grass, but now they are by a lake and the sun is reflecting in the lake. On the back of the picture I wrote,

"Life is made up of free and non-free elements. Aren't we lucky that there is no permanent self to carry foreword after this life is over? We are free to live our life as we want and discover how to integrate free and non-free elements."

## 4/29/97: Fog in the Bay

I took a break from my normal working day to walk by the water in Sausalito, meditate, and do some of the strengthening exercises for my immune system. I noticed that I could not see San Francisco, Berkeley or Oakland because of the fog, but Sausalito was clear. The meditation period was quite nice, and I felt rather good to be doing the stretches again.

My surgery has been changed to 7:30 A. M. on Friday, May 9 and Julie Motz will attend!

In my session, today, with Leslie Davenport, I dealt with the anxiety I feel about the question of whether or not there is still cancer in my body that represents a threat to my life. She felt confident that this was a good session for more EMDR (Eye Movement Desensitization and Reprocessing), and I thought it wise to allow her intuition to guide our work together. Several issues came up with regard to various stances about my current physical condition. The issues that were most prominent in my mind were the unattractiveness of radical cystectomy on the one hand, and the powerful healing session I had with Leslie on March 21 on the other. I needed to break through my resistance to allow the radical cystectomy to be part of my healing, and not seeing it as an invalidation of "healthy cells grow all by themselves." In the end, I realized that I was doing my best to help my recovery, and that as long as I kept looking deeply into alternatives as they come to me, I don't have to feel bad about anything I've done. It is this attitude that brought Julie Motz into my surgery, and gave me the opportunity to see Don Alejandro.

In the evening, I attended the "Life Threatened" group at the Center for Attitudinal Healing and my wife attended the "Care Givers" group. Our group was quite smaller than last week, and all but one person was there last week. It dawned on me how much worse off each of the other members were than me, and I was struck with a feeling of compassion for their suffering. When it was my turn to share, I offered a copy of *Yellow Stream* to the Center, and talked about Julie Motz. One of the people there had met her at the home where she is staying and said that she was pretty incredible. I believe her! I also spoke about Don Alejandro and my nervousness over next week's biopsy.

### 4/30/97: A View from the Waterfront

Today was a quiet day as far as cancer work is concerned. The only thing to report is that I took about an hour and a half out of my work day to walk by the bay, meditate, and do the immune system building exercises. All of these activities brought a nice, peaceful feeling, without the anxiety I was feeling yesterday about the surgery next week.

### 5/1/97: It's May, It's May!

I started the day off by taking the girls to school. From there I went to Cascade Falls in Mill Valley to do the immune system building exercises and meditated, but it was too cold to sit quietly that early in the morning. Nevertheless, I did the exercises and walked for about thirty minutes up on Mount Tamalpais, going uphill from the falls. The walk was very pleasant and I enjoyed it very much. I was able to maintain mindfulness most of the way.

The meeting at Cancerport was rather typical. I announced the Julie Motz lecture next week, and told everyone that she was going to be at my surgery. Other than that, all I had to report was my nervousness over the procedure next week.

Alan Sheets was gentle and caring. He is really interested in doing something about the pain in my knees. He wants me to videotape my tennis play so that he can see just why I'm wearing out the toes of my right shoe faster than any other part of the shoe.

At night, I went to my Evolutionary Circle group. Many people were feeling tired last night, especially me! Once again, the theme was laying on of the hands healing, and I was the first subject. The healing felt good. I remember one of the healers saying that I was surrounded by love and joy in my life! What a nice idea!

### 5/2/97: Your Average American Day

This morning I went in for my blood work for Dr. Belknap. In addition, I had blood taken for a nutritional analysis of my blood recommended by Dr. Rossman.

Later, I went to Leslie Davenport's group at Marin General Hospital. Leslie did a guided imagery which evoked the four elements. She began with the earth element by having us imaging our feet grounded to the earth even through our socks, shoes, the floor of the room, and on down through the building. She continued with the water, air, and fire, building on the images we had already constructed. Upon completion of the guided imagery, we drew a picture to represent our experience. My drawing incorporated all of the elements focusing on the room in which we were meeting. The building in which the room was looked more like a safe than a building, and I remarked that we were trying to create a "safe" space with our group. Everyone laughed! The group was also quite excited about Julie Motz!

When I got home, I needed to rest, as I was expecting a visit from my ex-wife. She is visiting our son from Israel and wanted to visit me. She arrived one hour late in a broken down car and was more or less forced to spend the night! She even invited me to go to Yosemite with my son and her!

### 5/3/97: A Day Without Cancer

I decided to forget about cancer today. I played tennis early in the morning and had a normal breakfast afterwards. I didn't make my smoothie or take any vitamins at all. In the late afternoon, we went to a movie and dinner with the Rossmans. I had a normal day without the preoccupations with cancer. I suppose it's healthy to do this once in a while, especially in light of the great question coming up on Friday!

### 5/4/97: Tennis Again!

I had difficulty sleeping last night because I went to bed too late. I had passed the point of good sleep while we were at the Rossmans, but, by the time I got in bed, the "good sleep" urge had passed. I decided to play tennis again anyway! After three sets, I went to the Tamalpais Fire Station for a pancake breakfast. Sarah Huang was there with her whole family. I was surprised to find out that her husband already knew about my surgery scheduled for Friday! They surely have become marvelous friends over the years. I'm really grateful for all of their help.

### 5/5/97: Having a Bad Day

I had a bad day today, which probably resulted from not enough good sleep. I worked for a while in the morning, and then tried to take a nap. Once again, I couldn't sleep, but the quite, restful mindfulness of breathing kept me from caving totally in.

In the afternoon, I went to see Alan Sheets for a Feldenkrais treatment. Alan's gentle hands and compassionate understanding were very helpful. He was purposefully trying to move me into point nine on the enneagram, as this is my so-called, "heart point." The heart point on the enneagram is the place that you tend to move towards in a secure life situation. It goes in the direction opposite to the arrows on the enneagram. For me, as a point six, the heart point is point nine. Point nine on the enneagram represents sloth with respect to spiritual growth and doing good things for yourself. I often find myself there when I am comfortable and relaxing with my children. Point nine is the point where love enters the enneagram. It is a point where well-adapted individuals remain peaceful without turning away from problems. The point in the direction of the arrows is known as the "stress point." For me, this is point three on the enneagram. Point three represents the over-achiever, which experience I've had many times in my life as I have tried to enhance my professional career. For more information on these and other points on the enneagram, please visit *The Enneagram in the Electronic Tradition*.

When I returned home from my appointment with Alan Sheets, I once again attempted to nap, with a similar result to the morning. I know what is bothering me, but that hasn't helped my sleeping situation. I am rather nervous about the results of my transurethral resection of the bladder tumor (TURBT) on Friday.

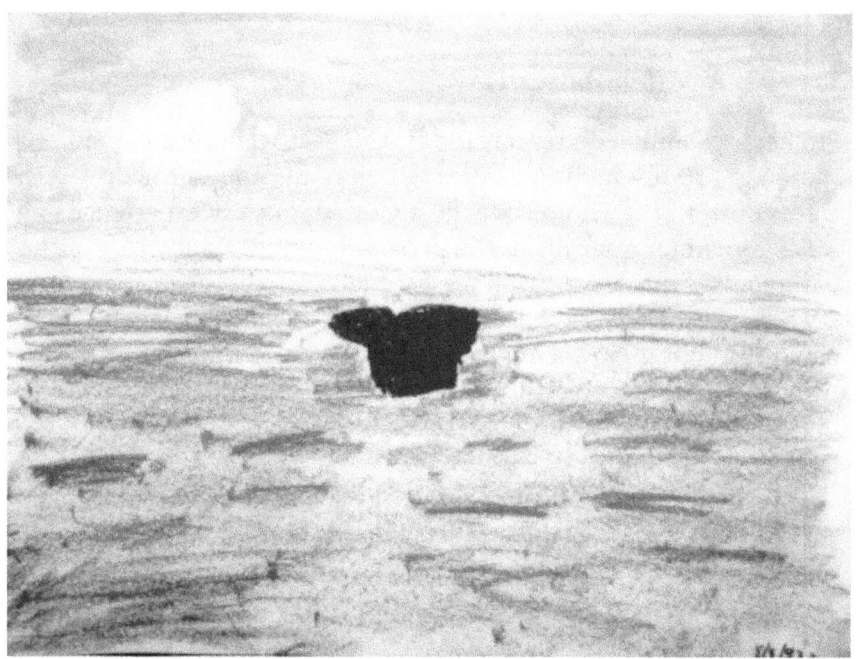

In the evening, I struggled to make it to Anna Halprin's class. She had just returned from the opening of the FDR Memorial in Washington, D. C. Apparently, her husband had a lot to do with the internal construction of the memorial. She sensed my discomfort and had us work primarily on our backs in order to conserve my energy. She had me moving my back in ways I've never experienced before, and it was quite amazing. I realized that one could do "moving meditation" in much the same way one does "walking meditation" in the Buddhist tradition. Her guided imagery took us to a clear blue sky above an expanse of ocean, with waves to match our breathing. We were to visualize a creature either in the sky or the ocean. I saw a whale most clearly and drew a picture of the wale just having completed a dive, with its tail still visible above the ocean surface. I wrote:

"I've created a 'whale' of a problem that needs to be solved. What I need to do is follow the lead of the whale and allow my tail *(how about tale - Yellow Stream!)* to float freely on the waves."

By the end of the evening, I was feeling much better. Anna placed me in the middle of the circle so that everyone could send me healing energy for the upcoming ordeal. Each person found a spot to touch me and bring even more healing energy into focus. It was a wonderful experience!

### 5/6/97: A Much Better Day

I'm having a much better day today, thanks to a decent amount of sleep (perhaps!) I worked in the morning before my appointment with Leslie Davenport. In the session, we did a guided imagery experience of what was happening in my life at the present moment. The threat of the pathologist finding cancer in my bladder was still the primary focus of my attention. Leslie, in her wisdom, asked me if there was a way that I could turn out good even if the results were not what I wanted.

Although I am still wrestling with this concept, I feel more confident in my ability to use my mindfulness to stay focused on all the good work I have done until now.

Next, I had to register for my surgery of Friday and make sure that everything was OK for Julie Motz. I didn't even have to wait, so I guess everything will flow smoothly on Friday.

Following my registration, I waited around for a neck and shoulder massage with Anna Pera at the Radiation Oncology Unit. It really felt great and came at a perfect time. I really allowed myself to relax into it and thus I got a lot of benefit from it.

In late afternoon, I had a complete physical with Dr. Belknap. The blood work was very normal and the rest of my health is surprisingly good! Dr. Belknap said with the blood tests and physical exam combined, he gave me an 80 to 90 percent chance of being free of cancer in my bladder! This information helped me to relax slightly.

At night, my wife and I went to the Center for Attitudinal Healing. Some people have been coming to the group for years, against which my three week barely measures up. However, I found it quite beneficial to speak once again about the dilemma I have with the outcome of my surgery on Friday. I am trying to hold either outcome as a part of my healing process, but I really, really prefer to be free of cancer now! I spoke a lot about my daughters' reaction to my illness and how they were such wonderful children. "We don't need a support group!" is what they always say! Their love and support is really helpful, even though I'm not quite sure that they know the worst case scenario.

### 5/7/97: Meeting Julie Motz

Julie is a sweet, lovely woman who really cares about people and their healing. I was immediately impressed by her softness and her energy. She seems to operate from a space of loving kindness and compassion.

After brief introductions, we got right down to the business of healing. Her theory is that cancer forms initially in the womb! The weak, unformed, incomplete cells develop there because of a lack of nutrients or in reaction to stress in the mother. The cells remain dormant until a stressful event triggers their erratic growth.

Well, I just wrote a beautiful piece about my experience with Julie Motz and Microsoft Word completely destroyed it after I completed the spell check! So, I'll do the best that I can to reproduce it.

The purpose of our meeting was to do two visualizations, one of my life from pre-conception to birth, and the other, a preview of the surgery on Friday. To get into the first, she had me breathe deeply several times and then had me imagine that I was breathing in through my naval, as this was the first place that I received oxygen in my body. I was then asked to experience what I was like just before conception. In my view, I experienced myself as empty of an individual existence, and therefore I was full of everything else. I was made up partly of my mother and partly of my father. I was also partly made up of their parents, and their parents...

At the moment of conception, I felt that I entered through the egg in my mother and was fertilized by the sperm. The tail of the sperm fell off just like a red leaf falls of a tree in autumn, after it has been nourishing the tree since it first grew in the spring. The tail of the sperm helped propel the sperm into the egg, which now flowed down to find a spot in the uterus. The single cell split into two, and the two into four, and so on. Soon, the cells started differentiating, and I was attached to the womb through the umbilical cord. It was through this chord that I obtain oxygen and nourishment from my mother. I also was bombarded with alcohol from Jewish observances and an occasional cigarette. Eventually, I grew to full term and emitted the hormones that indicated that I was ready to be born. I took my first breath of air and was cut off from my supply of nutrients.

The second imagery experience was shorter than the first. In the surgery preparation room, a nurse lovingly inserted the I. V. and gently rolled me into the operating room. Everyone there did their best to minimize the trauma I was experiencing, and I found myself waking up in the recovery room without much difficulty.

### 5/8/97: The Day Before

I got a massage from Elyse this morning. It was the best massage I ever had from her in probably two years of seeing her. Today, I seemed more relaxed and she was more able to penetrate my tissues. In addition, she has very healing hands and really cares about me. She spent a lot of time massaging my belly and bladder, and remarked how easy and free I was. It was a terrific experience!

Cancerport was once again very supportive to my surgery tomorrow. They were very encouraged by my report from Dr. Belknap, and excited by Julie Motz. Unfortunately, two of our members passed away this week. One of them was the lady I visited last month. Another member is having his last few days. I wonder where I stand in all of this.

In the evening, Julie Motz spoke at Marin General Hospital. After telling her story about how she became an energy healer, she spoke about the heart. She said that in Chinese medicine, the heart is the governor of the body, and that the seeds of emotion lie in different organs. She also said that anger is the energy of the heart. She talked about the pericardium, the protective tissue around the heart, as the location of the seat of love.

She gave her ideas about surgery, which essentially is that early trauma needs to be worked out through surgery. She also restated her proposition that cancer begins in the womb as immature, incomplete, fetal cells which stop growing and that wait around for an opportunity to grow out of control. In breast cancer, patients usually feel that their mother was burdened or embittered by the experience of mothering and this had an effect for the patient. Mothers were ambivalent or under a lot of stress during pregnancy.

She led us on a guided imagery experience through each chamber of the heart. The left aortic valve represents fear. The left ventricle valve represents anger, and is the origin of the heartbeat. The right aortic valve puts us in touch with pain, and the right ventricle is the origin of love.

### 5/9/97: An Angel Over My Shoulder

Today was the surgery and Julie Motz was the angel over my shoulder! She arrived at the hospital at 7:00 A.M. and stayed until about 9:30 or 10:00. I believe that Dr. Neuwirth appreciated her presence as well. I am not sure that I can tell you exactly what she contributed to the operating environment, but I felt comfortable. I haven't had a chance to find out what she thought yet, nor do I know the results of the biopsy.

The good news is that I was home by 3:00 P.M. and spent some real quality time with my son, who came to visit me. On the side that is not such good news is that I came home with a catheter in me, which has to be there until Monday to take pressure off of my bladder. Aside from feeling really tired, I'm doing quite well. I have no pain, and only a little discomfort from the catheter.

### 5/10/97: Recovery Day

Today I woke up with a headache and a sore throat. The sore throat is probably a result of the breathing apparatus during the surgery, but I can't explain the headache. I plan to spend much of the day in bed, watching the German Open Tennis matches. The phone has not stopped ringing this morning with well-wishers and friends!

### 5/11/97: Mother's Day

On my 56th birthday on October 8, 1995, my wife had just completed orthoscopic hip surgery six days earlier. As a result, she was not able to make much of a birthday celebration for me. In addition, my son's mother showed up just about dinner time with my son, so she wound up staying with us for takeout Chinese! It was one of the strangest birthdays I ever had! So, today, I'm the one who is unable to contribute to a Mother's Day celebration, although I did buy flowers and make a nice card on Thursday.

I imagine it will be another day of phone calls and visitors.

### 5/12/97: The Big Answer

Today, I was very nervous. I am supposed to have the catheter removed and receive the results of the biopsy this morning. I even spilled the catheter bag! I only have to wait another hour though.

Back from the surgeon! The preliminary biopsy report was NEGATIVE!

> *Breathing in,*
> *Breathing out,*
> *HEALTHY cells grow all by themselves!*
> *I am FREE of cancer!*

I have been ecstatic all day! A new perspective on combining alternative medicine with standard medical practice should be instituted nation-wide. This is a new theme for my work.

The complete biopsy report came in around 5:00 P. M. Although the results indicated that I had a complete response to the Shipley protocol, there was some new "transitional cell carcinoma, grade II/IV, without evidence of invasion."

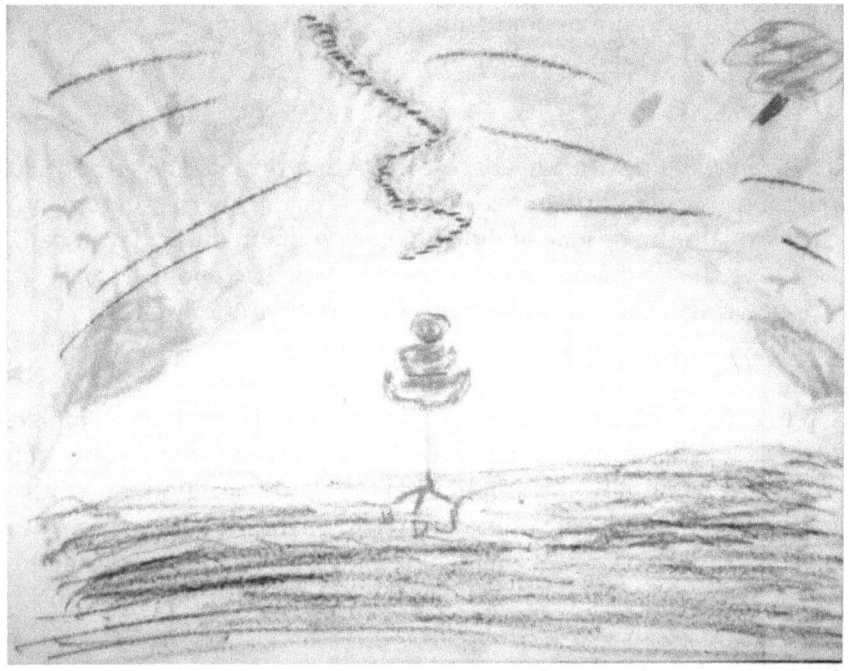

This means that my bladder is still susceptible to new growth, and I have to focus on prevention once the next round of chemo and radiation is complete. In essence, we continue with the bladder sparing protocol. This, in of itself, is quite a victory and cause for celebration.

So when I arrived at Anna Halprin's class, I was greeted with applause and cheers, and a spirit of celebration. After our usual round of checking in, we did some group movement, continuing the spirit of celebration. We followed this with more floor exercises from last week. Anna had us visualize a deeply relaxing spot in nature, and I immediately went to China Beach at Point Lobos State Reserve, near Carmel, California. The picture I drew was of this very spot. I wrote, "Guarding the sense gates - I can secure the future by mindfulness in the present."

## 10 - CONSOLIDATION TREATMENT

### 5/13/97: Free of Cancer!

My first appointment this morning was with Dr. Gullion. He was rather pleased that the induction phase of the Shipley protocol worked so well. He was also a little concerned about the 3 mm growth that was cut out of the surface of my bladder. He basically said that that was the nature of my bladder, and I would have to be watched. Nonetheless, we are still on the Shipley protocol and we begin chemotherapy and radiation next week. The basic protocol is the same, with chemo on Tuesday, Wednesday and Thursday with 5FU and cisplatin, and radiation twice a day on Tuesday and Thursday. The whole process repeats itself after a week off. Then I am finished with the protocol. I plan to call Shipley today to discuss the situation with him.

My next appointment was with Leslie Davenport. My major concern in speaking with her was about the 3 mm tumor that was removed. I am still confused about how it could be there, with treatments I've had so far, but now it is removed and my bladder is free of cancer. We worked on the sadness I felt as a result of having some cancer removed, and I connected it with a desire for intimacy, especially with my wife. I apparently still need to work out some personal problems having to do with asserting myself, while maintaining a close and intimate relationship with my wife.

To celebrate my recovery, T. R. took me lunch at Insalata in San Anselmo. We had a very nice lunch, followed by a stroll by Gelato and a chat in the park. T. is very grateful for my recovery and very inspired by it.

All afternoon I felt extremely tired. I suppose it was from too much running around on Monday and Tuesday. Therefore, I've decided to try to take it easy today.

I went to the Center for Attitudinal healing last night and shared my happy news. Everyone was happy for me, and I continued to express my mission of presenting alternative methods as something to be done in conjunction with convention medical practice. I shared the T-Up information with one of the patients who seems to be reaching the point of no return. This patient has a choice for surgery for which the recovery period could be as long as the remaining of his life if he doesn't have the surgery. The poor patient really has some tough decisions to make, and perhaps I can help him.

### 5/14/97: A Day of Recovery

I plan to spend most of the day working in bed today, as I really felt weak yesterday. I don't have any appointments I need to rush off to, but I am going to try some stretching exercises.

I spoke with Dr. Neuwirth today and found out for sure that the little 3 mm specimen was completely removed and there is nothing to worry about. Therefore, my bladder is totally **free** of cancer now, and I intend to keep it that way.

### 5/15/97: Another Day of Healing

I went to Cancerport this morning to share my good news and everyone was thrilled. Many people came up to me and told me that they were inspired by my success. Just about everyone wanted me to speak first, and I did. Naturally, I took the opportunity to share how important it was to combine conventional medicine with alternatives, and one of the members pointed out that they were no longer considered "alternatives," but "complimentary." All in all, I enjoyed the good wishes of everyone.

Next, I had the most incredible Feldenkrais session with G. T.. She had just completed a two and one half weeks of training. She worked mainly on my hips, pelvis, and shoulders, and I felt my body move in ways it never had before. Our contact in the session was extremely close and healing. I am most grateful for having these sessions with Gail. Next time, I'm also going to get a massage!

### 5/16/97: A Really Hot Day!

This morning, I slept until 9:00 A. M., which is very unusual for me. I needed the rest and felt all right about canceling my tennis date. Getting up so late almost made me late for Leslie Davenport's group. The hot weather kept the group quite small. When I shared about being free of cancer in my bladder, everyone was thrilled and inspired. This gave me the opportunity to express my feelings about integrative medicine, and I am beginning to think that I am preaching to the choir!

Leslie led us in a guided imagery experience that focused on qualities we would like to have in our beings. I focused on self-love, self-acceptance and joy. The experience was tremendously peaceful and

I had many moments of joy. When Leslie asked us to focus on our little circle, I was reminded of the *metta* or loving kindness blessings that I use so often. While the other people drew pictures of their guided imagery experience, I wrote out the *metta* blessings for each of the cancer patients in the group. This is what I wrote:

*May you be at peace!*
*May your heart remain open!*
*May you know the beauty and the radiance of your own true nature!*
*May you be healed!*

In the traditional way of practicing *metta*, as I was taught, one starts with showering loving kindness blessings on oneself, because if your heart isn't open, it's awfully difficult to reach another. Next, you proceed to shower the loving kindness blessings on someone you love or someone you are close with. This is to bring them joy and heal their pain. After that, you shower the loving kindness blessings on someone you are having a little difficulty with, in order to learn forgiveness and open your heart to the person who hurt you or with whom you are not communicating very well. Finally, you imagine the earth, floating like a jewel in the vast emptiness of space, with its green forests and fertile lands, white mountain tops, blue ocean, and brown deserts. You beam down loving kindness vibrations to all beings, and repeat the loving kindness blessings to all occupants of the earth. You end with, "May All Beings Be Happy!" The last statement has been my traditional screen saver for many years!

My daughter just got elected to the council at school and we are going to celebrate her victory and my recovery tonight at the Buckeye!

## 5/17/97: Laure's Bat Mitzvah

This morning we went to Laure's Bat Mitzvah. Like her sister years ahead of her, the job she did was extremely excellent! Every aspect of the service moved me. It was not a coincidence that the Bat Mitzvah was the first Shabbos after my biopsy report. This gave the rabbi the opportunity to "Bench Gomail," a blessing for those who have recovered from a serious illness. I felt moved and comfortable in being in synagogue with my family and friends.

The reception at night was at the Viansa Winery in Sonoma County. It was an amazing setting, overlooking a 90 acre wetlands sponsored by the winery. The food and dancing were superb, and I found myself relating quite well with the people at our table and others. It was great fun!

## 5/18/97: A Midsummer Night's Dream

My wife and I went to see a production of the ballet, "A Midsummer Night's Dream." Our friend's daughter danced the leading role and she looked like a professional. I was very moved by the performance as a whole.

Today, however, has been as sad day for me. I woke up feeling very vulnerable and emotional. I am a little afraid of the next round of chemotherapy and radiation, but besides that, I'm sad that my energy has not returned to its normal level. I feel physically and emotionally exhausted most of the time, even though everyone tells me how good I look. Having cancer is such a drag. I really need to pull myself together. Writing helps. Mindfulness helps, but I feel some underlying sadness now that is hard to deal with. It could be that I am just doing too much since the last surgery, but I keep thinking about my disappointments in life. I know that these feelings are impermanent and that I'll feel better soon. Maybe after dinner!

All day I had been thinking about Thich Nhat Hanh and how I've used mindfulness to keep calm. At one point, I was feeling that mindfulness had kept me alive, and I started to cry. I'm planning to attend a retreat with Thich Nhat Hanh in September in Santa Barbara. I explained all this to Dr. Rossman as we drove to a restaurant in Mill Valley. As we walked in, I looked over to the wall on my left and saw Reb Anderson, former abbot of Zen Center! I spoke with him briefly about my illness and about my mindfulness meditation. I had placed his name and that of the current abbot in my Wizard at the beginning of my illness, but I have never got around to calling either one! Now the word is out.

## 5/19/97: Conversation with the Rabbi!

This morning, Rabbi Nathan Siegel came by. We took a walk by the bay in Sausalito and talked about many things. When we arrived back at my house, we had "Jewish Penicillin" together. Then I found out that I had to have an X-Ray simulation run at 3:15. This conflicted with my oncology appointment, so I had to juggle the appointments.

The oncologist reported that my blood work was excellent and that everything was a "go" for chemotherapy tomorrow. The simulation turned out to be a simple taking of a few pictures and confirmation of the new blocks for the treatments tomorrow. They are going to irradiate a smaller area this time, and they had to verify all of the settings. The actual radiation dosage is less than before.

**5/20/97: Kunta Kinte Meets the Show Princess**

I began my consolidation phase of chemotherapy and radiation this morning. There were so many patients in oncology that it took until 10:00 for me to get hooked up. D. B. drove me to the oncology center and T. R. came later for a visit. T. mentioned again that his former girlfriend was marrying a six foot four South African. He said that this was a meeting of Kunta Kinte with the "Snow Princess!" For the most part, I was rather tired during the chemo, but I made it through without too much discomfort.

After my early afternoon radiation treatment, I met with Dr. Halberg. She is really nice, and spent the most unhurried time with me that I had experienced with any physician on my team since Dr. Torigoe spent almost two hours with us. She was caring and patient, even though she was interrupted several times to look at X-Rays, and other short tasks. I was rather surprised by her statement that she didn't expect me to have a complete response! She remarked that my initial invasive tumor was so aggressive and so extensive that she was surprised and happy by the pathology report! She also discussed the surface tumor with us, and said that she would not be surprised if I developed further surface tumors, and that anything we could do to prevent them was a step in the right direction. I had already told my wife that when this round of chemo and radiation was completed, I wanted to do a lot of new research on how to prevent bladder tumors from growing in the first place. Francine also mentioned that she was familiar with the anti-biotic trials at Pan Pacific Urology, but that I probably would not be eligible.

The second pass of radiation went without incident. I continued to do my visualization of the radiation as light entering my body and encouraging immature cells and potential cancer cells to shrivel up and be eliminated through my normal elimination channels. I also visualize my body as transparent to the radiation in such a way that the X-Rays affect the immature cells and potential cancer cells and then pass through my body, as in the X-Ray transmission studies in physics. I want to chat with the radiation physicist to understand the X-Ray transmission studies in more detail, as it has been almost thirty years since I left the field of physics for computers.

### 5/21/97: The Second Day of Chemo

Since there is no radiation today, the second day of chemo went rather smoothly. By 11:45, I was re-hydrating and all of the chemotherapy was in me. Now I just have to wait until all the saline solution flows through.

I'm a little tired today and a little bored. The files I downloaded from NGC yesterday put me no further into testing my code, as it didn't compile. I'll have to try that again today.

### 5/22/97: Blood Everywhere!

On this, the last day of chemo for this week, I had a small mishap. The tube from the i.v. broke free from the needle and blood started spilling all over the floor. It was rather scary, but in the end, it was quite harmless. Everything was put back without disturbing me too much, but I felt queasy the whole rest of the day.

I had two visitors at the oncology center. On was Jordy from Anna Halprin's class. She gave me an exceptional foot massage and we could have spent the whole day together. The other visitor was A. M., who had to walk over from her office because her car broke down. When we left the oncology center, my wife took her home in the city.

The rest of the day and the next were spent in recuperation. I'm still recovering from the third day of chemo.

### 5/25/97: More Down Time

I haven't written much in the past few days because I am still recovering from the last round of chemotherapy and radiation. I spend most of the days lying in bed, reading, and trying to maintain mindfulness. I feel a bit nauseous all the time. Some time I have tremendous gas pain, but most of the time, I just lie in bed and recover. It's not very exciting, but it sure beats the alternative of radical cystectomy!

### 5/26/97: One Memorial Day!

Today, I'm finally starting to feel better! The effects of the chemo seem less and I am in a better mood. I've been reading Timeless Healing by Dr. Herbert Benson, who is credited with discovering the "relaxation response." The book is aimed at convincing the medical profession that self-care should be an important part of healing, and that we all have "remembered wellness." He also points out the value of spiritual beliefs in terms of how quickly and how well someone can recover.

I have devoted much of the morning to my meditation practice, "healthy... free!" I seem to be able to keep the awareness of the in breath and the out breath in the background of my consciousness, even while sleeping (sometimes), but there seems to be something going on in the foreground that escapes my awareness. I notice the impermanence of the various thoughts and emotions as the pass through the foreground of my consciousness, but I'm not sure where this is supposed to lead.

### 5/27/97: Finally Feeling Better

I woke up twice this morning. The first time was to the sprinkler system in the back yard beginning to water the plants. The second time was when the phone rang. Now I am up and feeling better than I have for days.

During the night, I got some answers to the questions I raised yesterday about the foreground thoughts and feelings. I started thinking about what exactly was going on and I remembered two schools of thought about it.

The first school of thought comes from the teachings of the enneagram. In this school of thought, we function from three centers of intelligence: the physical or body center, the emotional center, and the intellectual center. These are also referred to as the belly, heart, and head center, respectively. Because we function from these three centers, we have bodily based experience impinging on our consciousness whenever we feel a slight pain or discomfort. We have an emotional experience whenever our feelings are triggered. Finally, and probably most of the time, we are bombarded through our mental center with thoughts, memories, plans, images, dreams (really another type of image), and so forth. In addition, we must note that energy follows attention. That is, wherever we place our attention, our energy will follow. If we are focused on a goal we want to accomplish, we may be able to place all of our attention on that goal.

We can actually create pretty much at will each of these experiences. For example, don't think of an elephant! What happened? You probably thought about an elephant and had an image of one in your mind. So basically, this is the content of the mind, according to the enneagram.

The Buddhist philosophy about these matters is surprisingly similar, although it doesn't deal with three centers of intelligence. In *The Art of Happiness*, Myrko Fryba talks about the four levels of experience on page 88:

Immediate experiencing of real events, processes, and states (and the feelings and sensations associated with them) bodily taking place in the present moment.

1. The bodily experienced meaning of represented (remembered) events, relations, constellations, situations, and scenes (and the feelings and sensations associated with them) that have led to current states of feeling and alterations of consciousness.
2. Conceptual thinking related to the flow of immediate experiencing or to the felt meaning of entire situations, which are presently happening. From this thinking are derived matrices and programs for apprehension and action (to the extent that they are consciously accessible and thus also "thinkable").
3. Conceptual thinking whose content has no relationship to the current state of the thinker and thus which has no conscious relationship to experiential reality. This could be a kind of non-reality-related babbling that is unconsciously motivated and directed, or mechanical data processing (for example, calculation), or it could also be wise reflection on rules and programs with the help of the meta-language of Abhidhammic algebra-in other words, planning and coordinating of liberational strategies. The key point here is that this level of experience has no present bodily anchoring in reality.

Later, when describing *Satipatthana-Vipassana* exercises, he refers to these as the four foundations of mindfulness:
1. Contemplation of the body (*kayanupassana*)
2. Contemplation of the feelings (*vedananupassana*)

3. Contemplation of consciousness (*cittanupassana*)
4. Contemplation of mental contents (*dhammanupassana*)

When practicing mindfulness meditation, one becomes aware of the different categories of experience and systematically assigns what I have called "foreground" material to one of the categories and returns to concentration on the object of mindfulness. If the experience is related to light, color, sound, noise, warmth, movement, trembling, itching, stinging, pressure, lightness, etc., it is assigned to the body. If the experience is pleasant, enjoyable, pleased, amused, bored, sadness, pain, indifference, etc., it is assigned to the feelings. If the experience is concentrated, scattered, tense, greedy, hate-filled, freed, etc., it is assigned to consciousness. Finally, if the experience is thinking, wishing, planning, intending, trust, doubt, knowledge, etc., it is assigned to mental contents. One tries to make the assignments as quickly as possible and return to the object of mindfulness.

My wife and I went to the Center for Attitudinal Healing together tonight. I went primarily because she wanted to go and I am not sleeping well, so I thought I'd go. I was deeply moved by the experiences shared by the members of the group! I felt compassion and understanding come to the foreground of my consciousness, and I realized that my side effects from chemotherapy and radiation are pretty slight compared to what some of the people are facing. I did a short sharing of my treatment plan, Dr. Halberg's surprise statement, and a few other things, but I got more out of listening deeply to other people.

## 5/28/97: Tea and Pumpkin Cake

This was the first day I felt almost normal! Lucky for that, too, because I had to go to Menlo Park to complete my performance evaluation with my boss. The day in Menlo Park was quite wonderful. The results of my review were acceptable except for one slight disagreement, which we are in the process of working out. Once the review was complete, we went to lunch, as we had done so many times before. Over all, we spent about two and one-half hours of quality time together, talking about business, raising girls, martial arts, and a variety of interesting topics.

In the evening, I went to the final class of Moving Towards Health with Anna Halprin at her studio in Kentfield. I had been to her studio once before about twenty-three years ago with Gabrielle Roth, and it was even more beautiful than I remembered. The night air was cool and comfortable and the setting in the woods was quite inspiring.

After a check in, in which I shared my progress report, we did some movements on the deck. We each walked around the deck for a while to find our "spot." Mine was at the East end of the deck facing West with a view of the very top of Mt. Tamalpais. It was gorgeous in the early evening sunlight. We made the movement into a ritual by performing the movement in each direction. Then each member was asked to dance their favorite movement and we did each person's movement in each of the four cardinal directions.

Next, we took a silent walk in the wood around her three acre estate. At a certain point, she asked us to fan out and find our "tree." We then spent about one-half hour with the tree, asking it questions, feeling its growth, and merging with "treeness." I picked a rather tall redwood, which I was willing to share with one of the other participants, but she marched off to find another tree. I embraced the tree, listened to its growth, and tried to encircle it with my arms, but it was too big. So instead, I walked around the tree, which was no easy task, since the tree was situated at the top of a two or three foot embankment. Towards the end of the time with the tree, I leaned on the tree with my back supported by the tree. It was a comfortable position to observe the connection, and it also allowed me see other elements in the environment. When the bell rang, and everyone headed back to the deck, I waited to the end and urinated on the tree. I had asked the tree if it minded the last vestiges of my disease being sprayed on its trunk, and the tree said that for decades all kinds of deer, rabbits, skunks, and other animals had done so and the tree felt nourished by each one. My act was a symbolic representation of cleansing the cancer and drugs from my system, as well as a way of claiming my territory in that little wood.

Back at the studio, we drew pictures of our excursion, and then danced what we drew before sharing our drawings. In the dance, Anna Halprin became my tree and supported my back while we moved together. Eventually, we encompassed the whole troop and focused our healing energies around a woman who was not fine when she arrived. It was a group hug embracing a lot of love, and it felt delightful.

My picture is shown below. It is called *Yellow Stream*, of all things! Note that all of the trees grow clearly past the top of the hillside and all of the little leaves, branches, and other natural elements that are part of the drawing. The tree is in separate from the other non-tree elements. In fact, the tree depends on the non-tree elements for its existence. It derives nourishment from the environment, and my contribution was minimal, if not symbolic. When I shared the meaning of my picture, everyone go hysterical. We had a good laugh for a long time.

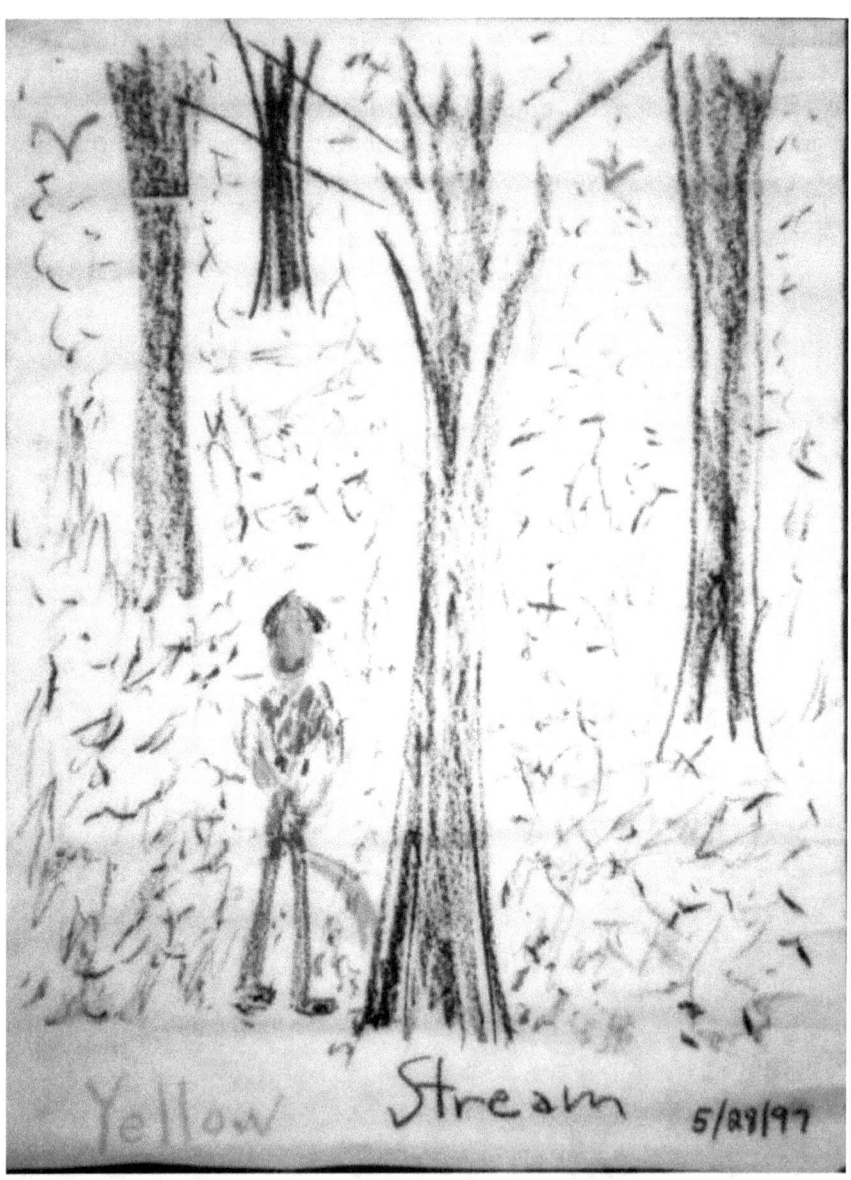

At the conclusion of the group, Anna invited us into her house for tea and pumpkin cake. This brought the spirit of the group together and we hung out for about another hour. I found myself swinging on a hammock with two women, two of my favorites. We talked about a lot of things and when I told them that I had an alternative title for the book, *Healthy Cells Grow All By Themselves*, one of them said rather enthusiastically, that she would buy a book with that name. Then I shared my image of "healthy cells grow all by themselves," and they felt even more comfortable with the title. So here we have it! The bound version of *Yellow Stream* will be hereafter called, *Healthy Cells Grow All By Themselves!* It's the official title now!

**5/29/97: Who Am I?**

I had a session with Leslie Davenport today. I went in with an agenda, which I promptly forgot. However, after rambling on about all the good things that were happening in my life, I finally remembered that I wanted to do a guided imagery in which all of the dead cells and unwanted drugs were cleansed from my system. The session was filled with ecstatic moments, as I saw little waterfalls cleanse and bring energy to my eyes and flow down to my abdomen, and breathed into various places in my body. We then did a body scan, and when we got to my bladder, she used my saying of "healthy cells grow all by themselves!" This, of course, triggered other ecstatic moments, and I channeled the wonderful energy right into my bladder. Then we went deeper into the process of going inward, and she suddenly came up with the question, "Who are you, Jerome?" I had an immediate flash of blue light come in through my belly center and could only answer, "When Bodhidharma was asked that question by King Wu, he said, 'I don't know,' and went off to meditate in a cave for nine years! So I don't know!" We went back into the guided imagery and a short while later she repeated the question. This time, my answer was the same, and I really got a kick out of it as if it were the real answer to the question. I felt like I had solved the koan quit well! The session ended soon after that, and I wanted to spend some more quality time with Leslie.

Later in the evening I went my Evolutionary Circle group. I spent a good deal of time explaining my physical condition, and everyone was thrilled. Then I began speaking about my spiritual state and invited them to follow the mindfulness path that I have been taking as an exercise. Everyone was enthusiastic about doing this, and the exercise lasted about twenty minutes.

I brought everyone into the breath in the belly by having them take several deep breaths, and then bringing their focus to the rising and falling of the breath in their bellies. I instructed them to repeat to themselves mentally, "healthy" with each inhalation, and to repeat "free" with each exhalation. At this point I let them get adjusted to what was going on internally with them before dealing with other objects of the mind. I then asked them to allow a physical sensation arise in their bodies and experience just what happens to their belly practice when the get lost in the effects of the body. After bringing them back to the belly breath, I instructed them on experiencing an emotion, so that they could experience what it was like to have some feelings while they were focusing on their breath in their bellies. I explained that energy follows attention and that if the emotion was strong enough, the breath observation practice would cease and they would get caught up in their feelings. I brought them back to the belly breath and guided them through the mental objects of thoughts, memories, plans, and images in the same way I had done the feelings, each time expressing the fact that the belly practice would dissipate if the energy in the thought, memory, plan, or image was strong enough to move their energy. Then I had them return the breath in the belly for a few moments of silence, just so they could experience whatever came into their consciousness.

Finally, I brought them back into the room and had everyone share their individual experiences. The experiment was a tremendous success and provided a setting for the rest of the group to check in. I told many other stories of my spiritual experiences since our last meeting, and felt tremendous love and support from the whole group. They are so happy that I am doing so well!

### 5/30/97: A Nothing Day!

I was supposed to have a Feldenkrais session and a massage from G. T. today, but she cut her finger and was unable to work. As a result, I did nothing but fight with my wife and work today! See, I'm really quite normal! Gail and I are scheduled to have lunch tomorrow at Kitty's place.

### 5/31/97: Suzanne's Birthday

To compensate for cutting her finger, G. T. agreed to meet me for lunch today at Kitty's Place. At least, this gave me the opportunity to tell her what was going on with me and to find out what her trip to Santa Barbara was like. After lunch, we took a nice walk in Fort Baker on Hawk Hill, where we saw magnificent views of San Francisco, the

Pacific Ocean, and Rodeo Beach. I was fairly exhausted from the effort, and decided to rest for a few hours.

During my rest period, I watched two documentaries on Tibet on PBS. The plight of the Tibetans is as bad as any people in exile. I felt like spending the $500.00 to attend a reception for the Dalai Lama that I was invited to on June 10, and I still may do so. When I was in India in 1975, I visited the village of Bodh Gaya, the location of the Bo Tree where Buddha became enlightened. There was one Tibetan restaurant there, and I ate there frequently. The people were so kind, even though one of the spoke very little English - just enough to allow me to order. There is a special beauty about the Tibetans I've met, and along with Thich Nhat Hanh, I consider the Dalai Lama the most influential Buddhists of our day. If anyone is interested in helping out the Tibetan cause, please let me know!

When the programs were over, I decided to go to Suzanne Schmidt's birthday party, which turned out to be very special. Instead of the usual shuffling around and trying to figure who to talk to, Suzanne told us a story about her life and two other women read pieces of their writings. I was touched by all of this, for I felt that each one of the women was more accomplished writers than I, and I had something to aspire to in my writing. I am not putting myself down; I'm recognizing the talent I saw last night.

## 6/1/97: J. and L. Return From Europe!

I got to play two sets of tennis at Eastwood Park! The gang was amazed that I was playing and I was playing so well. I had to rest a little during the second set, but, all in all, I did very well!

J. and L. came for lunch and we had a lovely time. Then I took my daughter to meet her friend to go to the circus and spoke to her father for a long time. We talked about my healing journey and his recent vacation. He was very happy for me and said that what I was doing was helping us all!

Later in the afternoon, I received an email message from Elisabeth Frauendorfer, Ph.D. about some new research she was doing about a theory about the cause and development of disease, and experiments leading to a possible therapy/cure. If anyone is interested in what she has to say, please send her email. I am planning to forward a copy to Michael Broffman to see what he has to say.

In the evening, R. C. came over with his daughter, daughter-in-law, and grandson for dinner. The daughter is graduating Marin Horizon School with my daughter, and they are close friends. R. C. is a self-made millionaire who we've been friends with since pre-school. His wife is on a two-week first-class tour of England, Prague, and Budapest for her 50th birthday. He's trying to sell his company now and feels really good about it. We spoke about a workshop he attended which called for speaking your own truth and not trying to change anyone else. The discussion was fascinating and could have gone on for hours. I'm sure we'll resume it the next time we get together.

**6/2/97: No Anna, No Dance!**

Today is Monday and Anna is not having class tonight. But I have to prepare for chemotherapy tomorrow morning. This involves having blood work done early this morning and a visit to Dr. Gullion at 10:00. So I arrived at Meris Labs at 9:15 A. M., and thankfully, I had my lap top with me so that I could get some work done. I didn't get to see Dr. Gullion until 11:15!

We discussed the protocol and my blood tests. He thought that in my situation, it was a good choice and he wished more bladder cancer patients consulted him before they had a radical cystectomy, so that at least a bladder sparing protocol could be attempted. Although my white blood count was the lowest they had tracked, it does not inhibit continuing the protocol. So, tomorrow, we start again, but for the last time.

**6/3/97 "There's Always Things We Can Do"**

I started chemotherapy and radiation again today and it was "no piece of cake" (tomorrow is my brother's birthday!). I had to be stuck four times before the i. v. took. In addition, the oncology group seemed to ignore the request of the radiation group that I be downstairs for my first radiation treatment by 12:30. So, Dr. Gullion cleverly sped up the protocol to grant their request, and I don't know if this is good or bad, so I won't pass judgment on it right now.

I was fairly wiped out after the chemotherapy and listened to a tape of Helen Palmer. There was so much good material in the tape that I easily fell asleep two or three times! I guess I'll try to use this tape rather than sleeping pills. Someday, I'll write more about what's on the tape.

L. C. took me to the second dose of radiation. During our trip in the rush hour traffic, I was telling him about my daughter's paper, <u>Zen Buddhism: Its Beliefs and Effects on Society</u>, which she is presenting tomorrow night. In spite of my so-called weakness from the chemotherapy, I experienced that her opening statement,

> *"A special transmission outside the Scriptures;*
> *No dependence upon words and letters;*
> *Direct pointing to the soul of man;*
> *Seeing into one's own nature."*

was true and felt a wave of ecstasy move through my body and focus on my bladder.

My wife really needed to go to the "Care Givers'" group at the Center for Attitudinal Healing tonight, so I went to the "Life Threatened" group. It was the best experience I ever had at the Center! I was moved so much by many of the opening statements that I felt the desire to speak first. I shared the difficulties that I was experiencing with my wife, and then the beautiful experience I had at Anna Halprin's studio last week. Then I told the group about the email I sent to the Dalai Lama, which I quote here:

Dear Your Holiness:

> I have been a practicing Buddhist since 1985. I have been invited to the Tibet House Reception at the home of Ingrid and Reuben Hills in San Francisco next week, but I am unable to attend because I am recovering from bladder cancer and the requested donation is a little too steep for me. However, I have inspired many of my wealthier friends to donate to Tibet House.
>
> If I were to attend, I would ask you the following question: I know that Padmasambhava is known to have said, "When the iron bird flies and horses run on wheels, the Tibetan people will be scattered like ants across the world and the Dharma will come to the land of the Red Man!"
>
> I want to know, first of all, how authentic is this quote? Secondly, I want know how he could have foreseen ALL of these developments back in 828 A. D.?
>
> Thank you so much for your response. If you have time, you may want to visit my web site, http://mountainsangha.org to see just how much mindfulness meant to me on my healing journey.
>
> I love you and adore the Tibetans I've met. In 1975, I visited Bodh

Gaya and the Bo Tree of the Tathagata!

Thank you so much.

I raised the same questions with the group and everyone was touched! I also shared my experience in the car on the way to radiation therapy.

The other members shared so much valuable experience that I felt honored to be there. Because of the guiding principles of the Center, I feel bound not to reveal their stories except to say that one member's significant other had made the above statement when news that was not so good was revealed. I offered that member and two other members who touched me deeply by their stories to do guided imagery with them if they wanted. In addition, since the Center is having financial difficulties, I felt moved to offer a workshop called, "Zen and the Art of Healing," with all proceeds going to the Center. The two facilitators I spoke with about the workshop were wonderfully supportive! At the end of the group, I passed on the healing stone I received from Anna Halprin and passed around the group at the Center to one of the participants who I felt needed it more than I. The person was extremely grateful and said, "Do you mean I can keep it?"

## 6/4/97: The True Teaching of Zen

The second round of chemotherapy went without incident. I chose to spend the day in an examination room with a hospital bed to try to get some sleep. I also broke may lap top and have to send it to Nashua, NH to be repaired. The tapes I brought to listen to were quite suitable for my purpose of getting some rest.

In the evening, I barely made it to my daughters' presentations on the culture of Japan. My twelve-year-old demonstrated the making of Sushi and prepared an exhibit of other Japanese foods. My fourteen-year-old gave a speech on <u>Zen Buddhism: Its Beliefs and Effects on Society</u>. I was so proud of both girls, but I had to leave early to get in bed.

## 6/5/97: The Last Day of Treatment!

Today, I complete the Shipley bladder sparing protocol. Once again, I choose to spend the day resting in the examination room. It was uneventful, except for the lovely visit of A. M. Now it's time to get in bed again until my final radiation treatment at 5:00 P.M. Then it's time to celebrate, but I won't do so until I recover from the chemotherapy and radiation. When I completed that last radiation treatment, I received a diploma for a job well done signed by all of the staff, but not the doctors.

I gave Dr. Gullion and Dr. Halberg copies of *Yellow Stream* and asked for their comments about the protocol and my response to it. If their writings are not too delayed and contain some valuable information, I'd like to include them as an appendix to *Yellow Stream*.

## 11 - RIDING THE BULL HOME
### 6/6/97: The 10 Bulls of Zen

After the ordeal I had this week, I finally feel that the disease in under control, even though I don't have all of my energy back. The situation reminded me of the Ten Bulls of Zen, by Hakuan, transcribed by Nyogen Senzaki and Paul Reps, illustrated by Tomikichiro Tokuriki, HTML version by Jamie Andrews.

In these pictures, the bulls represent the eternal principle of life, that is, truth in action. Each bull represents a step in the direct experience and realization of one's true nature. Riding the bull home, or "coming home on the Ox's back" was traditionally the sixth bull of Zen. This is what Hakuan had to say in D. T. Suzuki's, *Manual of Zen Buddhism* (Grove Press, New York, 1960, page 132):

> *The struggle is over; the man is no more concerned with gain and loss. He hums a rustic tune of the woodman, he sings simple songs of the village boy. Saddling himself on the ox's back, his eyes are fixed on things not of the earth, earthy. Even if he is called, he will not turn his head; however enticed he will no more be kept back.*

and the poem:
> *Riding on the animal, he leisurely wends his way home;*
> *Enveloped in the evening mist, how tunefully the flute vanishes away!*
> *Singing a ditty, beating time, his heart is filled with a joy indescribable!*
> *That he is now one of those who know, need it be told?*

I'm writing this detail to express a feeling of having tamed my disease. Not that it won't have to be monitored from time to time, but the major danger is over, and I feel joyous!

Although the web site will continue to grow, this will be the last chapter in the book, *Healthy Cells Grow All By Themselves*, as I will submit *Yellow Stream* for publication as of Father's Day, June 15. I feel that this is an important time for me to release the book because my children should be quite secure that the worst part of my disease has been conquered by then, and it is a good day to celebrate! The book will conclude with a chapter that summarizes and prioritizes my healing process, and should be very interesting.

### 6/9/97: One Bite at a Time, One Step at a Time

The last few days have been really rough on me. The chemotherapy and radiation are really taking their toll on me in a big way. I haven't even been able to compute these last few days!

I've had bladder spasms, diarrhea, and gas pains on three successive days, accompanied with tremendous exhaustion. I spend most of my days lying in bed and practicing mindfulness of breathing. I have read a little, listened to a few tapes, and watched the French Open, but most of time, I just lie in bed. Breathing in, "healthy cells grow all by themselves." Breathing out, "I'm free of cancer!"

When it comes to eating and moving, I find that I can only eat one bite at a time! When I walk, I can only take one step at a time. Of course, this is normal behavior, but in my present physical state, there seems to be awareness at a different level of each bite, of each step.

### 6/10/97: Another Step

Today was a little better than yesterday and the day before, but I didn't feel well enough to go to the Center for Attitudinal Healing, as my wife did. I worked part of the day, and sent a manuscript of Healthy Cells Grow All By Themselves. I think this effort was a little too much for me, so I spent the rest of the day in bed, mostly following my breathing, but I did listen to the tape of my session with Leslie Davenport from May 29 again. I still don't know who I am or where I am going! I know that I want to spread the word about self-healing and remembered wellness as far as possible. If that's what I'm supposed to do, so be it!

I continue my mindfulness meditation as often as possible, coupled with frequent imagery sessions about healing my bladder. I've begun to re-read *The Heart of Buddhist Meditation* by Nyanaponika Thera to support my mindfulness practice. I highly recommend it!

### 6/11/97: My First Outing

Today I was feeling well enough to have lunch at Kitty's Place with my wife and J. C. We had a lovely lunch, and I felt good to be out. I then got a haircut for my daughter's graduation on Friday. Now I'm ready for another rest! This has been a really difficult time for me, but I try to keep it together with mindfulness meditation and "mind stories."

## 6/12/97: "Let My Heart Fly Open, Let Me Come To You"

I was speaking with Joe, one of the facilitators of the Life Threatened group at the Center for Attitudinal healing the day before yesterday to find out what went on in the group. There was one person who wasn't given much of a chance of returning, and yet she did. I had been thinking about her the whole time I've been recovering from the treatment, and couldn't wait to talk to Joe about the person. As we were speaking, Joe told me the story of his illness and work with the Center, which I can't repeat here, except to say that he had had an experience of moving out of himself to the other.

Helen Palmer speaks about a similar experience. Our first line of work in the enneagram is to know ourselves. This we do through self-observation practice which corresponds quite closely with mindfulness meditation that I often write about. In fact, the self-observation practice that Helen teaches is to pay full attention to the breath in the belly, following the inhalation, the pause, the exhalation, and the return. This is the full cycle of the breath in the belly. As bodily sensations, feelings, thoughts, plans, memories, and fantasies enter into the mind, they are swiftly moved away, like a fallen leaf drifts slowly down by the effect of the wind. She teaches that when one becomes still in this way, one begins to get feelings that come before you know what you will feel, and that these feelings can be of the other. This process leads to the second line of work, which is to know the other as they know themselves.

When I spoke about similar matters with Leslie Davenport at our last session on May 29, I asked her what she thought was going on with me. She said that in Sufi terms, she felt that I was changing "*macoms*," which she described as "place." I had heard about *macoms* at the First International Enneagram Conference three years ago, but I still don't know much about them. She had said that one man's macom is another man's ecstasy. Apparently, as one moves from *macom* to *macom*, one becomes closer to the divine. My interpretation is that I am experiencing a great opening of my heart, which probably began in the spring and was furthered by my experience at Anna Halprin's studio on May 28.

The quote in the title is from a Sufi song that cries out for the presence of the divine. From this sparse information, I gathered that

Leslie thought that I was moving into a new state. In this state, I personally feel a transformation from thinking mostly about myself to thinking about others. I've always thought a lot about my children and my spouse, but now I am thinking about other people a lot, especially the ones in my support groups.

So, today, when I had a massage, followed by a Feldenkrais session with G. T., I could only think of this song. Her loving hands seemed to strip the chemotherapy of its grip on my healthy cells and, as she massaged my feet, I felt the unwanted cells leaving my body through my shoulders. Her work on my lower back, shoulders and abdomen was the best massage I've ever had in those particular areas. I felt so cleansed by the whole massage that I began to cry when I sat up to change over to the Feldenkrais lesson. My heart was singing, "Let my heart fly open, let me come to you!" I had never cried before after a massage, and I had never felt so touched by the divine. I'll never forget those feelings. It was like yearning for the divine and receiving grace. Throughout out my whole emotional experience, Gail was there with me with her loving presence and guided me to a safe space for us to continue with the Feldenkrais work.

The Feldenkrais lesson was shortened, due to the length of the massage, but it was excellent. She worked on my shoulders and my spine, and I really felt great! Then I gave Gail a shortened version of a Zero Balancing treatment, which I think she enjoyed. Nonetheless, it's up to her to write about it!

**6/13/97: "Let My Heart Fly Open, Let Me Come To You"**

The original title for today was, "Graduation Day," but after the events of the day, you'll see why I chose the same title as yesterday. It was another day of tremendous heart opening! Blessed be!

Twelve years ago, when my oldest daughter (R.) was almost two and one-half, and my youngest daughter (J.) was ten months old, I attended, almost reluctantly, the moving on and graduation ceremonies for Marin Horizon School. R. was just a toddler, and J. and infant, but my wife (M.) insisted that we go to the graduation "to support the school." So I put on my tie and sat in an uncomfortable folding chair for almost two hours. But something remarkable happened at the graduation. The graduating eighth graders each delivered a speech of gratitude and thanksgiving to their teachers, friends, and family. Each teenager expressed a feeling of confidence and spoke of their individual experiences attending the school. Each talk was so well organized and so moving that you thought you were listening to a high school valedictorian address. I'm telling you, I was truly impressed and amazed. I sat there and decided then and there that I wanted my children to grow up with such confidence, such a sense of individuality, such as sense of self-esteem, and such a love for learning that I was willing to sacrifice financially whatever it took to see them deliver their graduation addresses.

Well, today my dream came true! R. delivered the most emotional and moving speech I had ever heard! She spoke about individuality:

> "As President John Quincy Adams once said, "Individual liberty is individual power, and as the power of a community is a mass compound of individual power." And this is the true power of Marin Horizon School. I have experienced this for more than twelve years. Tenacious, patient, and understanding, these are the characteristics that Marin Horizon has helped me become. There are many great qualities of Marin Horizon, but the one that stands out the most is how each student is considered and individual."

Then she began to share some of her priceless memories from Marin Horizon School, and spoke about her closest friends. You can't imagine how much love these five girls have developed for each other over! And each young woman that spoke after her had much the same to say about the value and meaning of their friendship with R. As she was thanking her friends, tears started to swell up in her and everyone else who attended the ceremony. She thanked her teachers and the adults in her life, mainly our friends and the parents of the closest friends. Everyone was moved to tears.

Then she thanked her sister, and people wept more! You cannot imagine the love these two siblings have for each other. They have always been close, from the very beginning, and I feel that the way we brought J. into the family had a lot to do with it. When R. was still very young, we would speak to her about another child coming into the family soon, and that she would be loved even more because of her new sibling. The girls have always been close.

Next she thanked her mom for all the love and support, and this is what she had to say about me:

> "Last, but not least, my father, you have always been there for me

*even if you were going through rough times. You are so loving. You are the best father. I love you so much!"*

As she was speaking these words, my heart flew open, and I felt the divine presence as I wept for joy! You have to imagine the scene. There we were in a church in Mill Valley, and R. was at the podium looking more beautiful than you can imagine, with tear in her eyes and love in her heart. There wasn't a dry eye in the crowd! I'm telling you, this young woman looked so awesome that it made you wonder, "When did you become such a beauty?" Yes, truly, "let my heart fly open, let me come to you!"

After the ceremony, the kids went off on their own separate ways and M. and I went to celebrate with the parents of three of her best friends, as we have done for many years at the Buckeye Restaurant. We had such a joyous time! I ate the wrong things and drank too many sips of champagne, but it was worth it! When I had to leave early, each person stood up, hugged me, and kissed me and told me how much they loved me, and told me what a wonderful job I did in raising my children. I was so touched that I cried all the way home and continued to cry until M. came home. I am still having spontaneous fits of crying, as I write today's entry.

## 6/14/97: How Much Love Does It Take?

Today I went to a benefit concert of classical music for my friend J. W., a long-time friend and member of my small enneagram group. She is also living with cancer, and the Diamond Heart group she belongs to sponsored the concert. The concert raised more than $1,400 to help J. pay for her medical expenses. She's a great lady and deserves all the help she can get. There were more than fifty people there and I thought to myself, "How much love does it take to heal from cancer and get on with your life? How much love does it take to make you realize that you need to love yourself first, and then you can share it with others?" J. certainly was surrounded by people who loved her, and she was radiant!

I sat with D. K., another member of my enneagram group, and his wife. All three were so supportive of my situation, and when I had to lie down for the second half of the concert, D. was rubbing my feet!

## 6/15/97: Father's Day

Today is the last installment of Yellow Stream for the book, Healthy Cells Grow All By Themselves. I think it is appropriate to end the paper version here for several reasons. First of all, I'm finally on my way to recovery from the last effects of the chemotherapy and the radiation. Secondly, the book is dedicated to my children and my spouse, and what better time to end than on Father's Day? Thirdly, I want to share with you some of the secrets that I have learned in raising happy and independent children over the last twenty-eight years. While I still have young ones in the house (R. is fourteen and J. is twelve), my son is 28, and living a happy and independent life. And finally, I feel that my greatest accomplishment in life so far has been being a "dad" and raising such fine children. If other children were raised with the values and love that I have given to my children, things would be a lot better in the world.

So, what are my ideas about raising children? Well, one of the first things to think about is that

> *"Your children are not your children.*
> *They are the sons and daughters of Life's longing for itself.*
> *They come through you but not from you,*
> *And though they are with you yet they belong not to you.*
> *You may give them love but not your thoughts,*
> *For they have their own thoughts.*
> *You may house their bodies but not their souls,*
> *For their souls dwell in the house of tomorrow, which you cannot visit, not even in your dreams.*
> *You may strive to be like them, but seek not to make them like you.*
> *For life goes not backward nor tarries with yesterday.*
> *You are the bows from which your children as living arrows are sent forth.*
> *The archer sees the mark upon the path of the infinite, and He bends you with His might that His arrows my go swift and far.*
> *Let your bending in the archer's hand be for gladness;*
> *For even as He loves the arrow that flies, so He loves also the bow that is stable."*

This quote is from Kahlil Gibran, *The Prophet*, Alfred A. Knopf, New York, 1951. You have all probably read it before, but lost sight of the "arrow." I have always tried to keep in mind that my children have come through me, but not from me. I have also tried to remember that they have their own thoughts and dreams, which I cannot even imagine. I have always tried to give them the space to grow into special individuals, and, as you can see from R.'s speech the other day, it seems to be working.

I also value instilling upon my children the importance of developing a love for learning, and, as a result, have invested my hard-earned money on private education for all three of them. My son went to Mt. Tam Primary School, and the Branson School, each a fine independent school in their own right, before graduating from Stanford University. R. and J. have been in Marin Horizon School since they were about two years old! This school is based on Montessori methods, and fosters individuality, along with a respect for all life forms and other people's property. I love the education my daughters have received, and I feel that they are prepared for any eventuality.

Another area of parental concern is that of control, partly for the safety of the child, and partly for setting limits. In this area, I have always remembered what Shunryu Suzuki-roshi had to say about control in *Zen Mind, Beginner's Mind* (Waterhill, New York, 1970, p 32):

> "...Even though you try to put some people under some control, it is impossible. You cannot do it. The best way to control people is to encourage them to be mischievous. Then they will be in control in its wider sense. To give your sheep or cow a large, spacious meadow is the way to control him. So it is with people; first let them do what they want, and watch them. This is the best policy. To ignore them is not good; that is the worst policy. The second worst is trying to control them. The best one is to watch them, just to watch them, without trying to control them."

I was deeply affected by this passage back in the seventies when I first read it. I remembered it and applied it to controlling my children. This way, they had a "spacious meadow" in which to explore life and learn the boundaries that were set for them in a happy and contented way.

Among the other values I try to instill in my children is the ability to make decisions for themselves. To do this, I taught them a reliable subjective basis for making moral and ethical decisions based on clear comprehension of the alternatives. Included in this reliable subjective basis was a love and respect for all life forms and respect for other people's property, as mentioned before. As an example, when my son was eleven or twelve, he excelled in two activities that both made us proud. He was an excellent gymnast and a talented member of the San Francisco Boys Chorus. The gym was in San Rafael, and the Boys Chorus was in San Francisco, both more than ten miles from our house in opposite directions. We sat down with him when we realized that these activities were not only stressing us out, but causing him some concern. After weighing all sides of the issues, he decided to stay with the Boys Chorus. This was a momentous decision for him, as it led him into a direction of the performing arts. For example, at the Branson School, he played Biff in *West Side Story*, El Gayo in *The Fantastics*, and was one of the founding members of the Barber Shop Quartet. At Stanford University, while he minored in music, he was a member of the Stanford Fleet Street Singers, and director for two of his four years there. Since his graduation he has played major parts in *Iolanthe, La Boheme*, and *Naughty Marietta*. He plans to move to New York in August to try to make it into the big time, all the while maintaining his skill as a computer graphic designer. You can see some of his work by browsing to his web site, http:// http://micahfreedman.com/. And remember the he is a cancer survivor!

Well, enough of my ideas for raising children for now! What about the events and feelings of the day?

We were invited to lunch at Mikayla's by our friend J. and R., who own the place. J.'s sister was also there with her family. She and R. both studied with Anna Halprin, so we had many interesting conversations about various topics. Besides that, the food was magnificent and we had a difficult time leaving.

My son came back to the house and we spoke for hours. It was during this time that he revealed to me his plan to give New York a try. I was totally supportive, for I believe that he is still young enough to give it his all, and he always has the fallback position of doing computer graphics. What impact this will have on his almost seven year relationship with his girlfriend, I don't know and won't even try to predict.

## 12 – WHERE DO WE GO FROM HERE?

### 6/16/97: The Major Factor is Mindfulness

This morning, I went to a Feldenkrais class taught by Joanne at D. B.'s house. I've been there before, and always enjoyed it. Today was special because the lesson involved the knees and hips, which have been a problem for me over the past few years. G. T. treated me to lunch and we walked a little in Belvedere Park. I almost had my strength back.

The rest of the day I spent working on some new problems in the Sniffer. When will they ever end?

I was beginning to wonder, "Where do we go from here?" The treatments are done, but I am aware that surface tumors can recur under normal circumstances. My job is to continue to keep my circumstances on a higher plane. I have to keep on taking my supplements; continue with support groups, guided imagery, exercise, and body work. I should be back playing tennis by the end of the week! Nonetheless, the major factor is still mindfulness!

### 6/17/97: The Tail of the Kite

Today was one of those days that started out being very stressful, as I was under pressure to solve a bug and chauffeur my kid around, and it also ended with a lot of stress as a result of negative thoughts that entered my mind after attending the Center for Attitudinal Healing.

After delivering my daughter to the shopping center with her friend, I went for another healing massage with G. T.. She worked quite diligently on my shoulders and abdomen, and remarked that the effects of the chemo seemed much less. I also felt a strong healing coming into my body as she massaged my abdomen in a tender and loving way. This was the first time I had a massage at her house and we sat down for sushi afterwards. So I was feeling pretty good when I left her.

From there, I went to a session with Leslie Davenport. As I brought her up to date with all the wonderful experiences I've been having since our last session, I began to cry again, as the full extent of the emotional impact of the events hit me again. We talked at length about the opening of my heart chakra. During the guided imagery, she was trying to ground the energy so that my heart would stay open. While I was there, it seemed to work, but when I got home, I really experienced the fear of being hurt when I was so vulnerable. I spoke with her later on the phone and expressed my fears. To this, she once again emphasized the importance of grounding the energy rather than closing off.

All of these experiences led me to go the Center for Attitudinal Healing, even though my wife was taking the night off. At the Center, I shared the heart-warming events since last Thursday, and felt good about being open again. But then someone shared some experiences that made me start to think again, and I became lost in the fear. I began to doubt my love for myself, as I had most of my life. I felt like I was about to lose it and then the session was over and I could retreat into myself. I tried to explain what was going on to my wife, but wasn't able to compete with the TV.

So what started out stressful due to performance and duty wound up stressful due to fear and doubt. All of these characteristics can be explained through knowledge of my point on the enneagram. Point six, as I've mentioned before is the position of the doubter, and fear is the passion. It looks like I've allowed my old personality to rear up again in the face of stress. And then I wonder how I can alter my path of recovery so I don't wind up in the same place I was when the cancer struck. If I do, there will be no real healing, as I must heal my aching heart.

## 6/18/97: Eating Soup with a Fork

Today was probably the worst day that I've had since I received my diagnosis. I was full of emotion and frequently broke down crying. The morning was especially trying, as I was desperately trying to get in to see Leslie Davenport, having told my boss that I wouldn't make it in today. The best she could offer was 6:00 tomorrow evening, so I jumped on it.

The doubt factor was the strongest. I doubted myself. I doubted my recovery. I was consumed by the idea that if things didn't change in my life, I would have more trouble as a person who had had cancer than a person that has cancer and knows it. I was extremely afraid to be hurt and abandoned. Now that I am well, are my friends still going to care about me? Will I be able to continue to create my dream? Will my heart remain open? Or, is it already out to lunch? What about the divine love I was feeling last week? What about the love my daughter expressed for me last Friday? How can all of this be simultaneously true in my experience?

Well, here I am, eating soup with a fork! You'll have to read *It's Easier Than You Think* by Sylvia Boorstein to get the full impact of what I'm doing! The book is about the Buddhist way to happiness, and I spent the afternoon reading the whole thing, in between fits of tears and meditation. One of the main ideas that struck me from the book was that, "Traditional Buddhist texts teach that the ability to sustain attention in the truth of the moment is the antidote for doubt." Many of her stories also moved me to tears. One of the bells of mindfulness that happened during my meditation was as call from a member of Anna Halprin's group who offered to give me a massage tomorrow after talk at Voices of Healing.

I guess I'm doing a little better now that I'm eating my soup with a fork and writing in Yellow Stream!

## 6/19/97: Voices of Healing

I woke up this morning feeling a lot better than yesterday. I had spent much of the night doing mind stories and metta meditation. The metta meditation is a loving kindness meditation from the Buddhist tradition. I've adopted mine from several sources and it goes like this:

First you shower yourself with loving kindness by saying to yourself with feeling:

*May I be at peace.*
*May my heart remain open.*
*May I know the beauty and the radiance of my own Buddha-nature.*
*May I be healed.*
*May I be happy, truly happy!*
*May I not cause anyone to suffer.*

Then you shower the loving kindness blessings on someone you love, substituting "you" for "I" in the above rendition. You then shower loving kindness blessings on someone you are having a problem with and follow with showering loving kindness blessings on the whole world, imagining the earth floating in the vast emptiness of space. I practiced this meditation for several hours and woke up feeling fine! It was really important to shower the loving kindness blessings on myself first, so I could feel good enough about myself to shower the blessings on my spouse and other people I love in my life.

In the afternoon, I went to a meeting of Voices of Healing in Mill

Valley. It turned out to be a support group much like the life threatened group at the Center for Attitudinal Healing. I was touched by people's healing stories.

After the meeting, I received a massage from Pauline from Anna Halprin's group, and I've added her name to the resources list. Pauline is also living with cancer and continues to study with Gabrielle Roth. She was gentle and prayerful as she gave me an Eselan massage. The massage was excellent, and the mood was enhanced by the Tibetan music in the background.

From there I went to a session with Leslie Davenport. I needed to see her again this week because I felt in crisis with the thought of resuming my life as it was prior to the cancer. I felt and still feel that if I allow those conditions to be re-established, I'd be really susceptible to a recurrence of my disease, and this made me panic. There were other issues that came up, especially how much love if flowing into my life from many sources, but I was in the middle of a severe doubt attack.

### 6/20/97: A Scare in the Night

In the middle of the night last night I woke up from a dream and I was lying on my left side. I noticed a somewhat painful feeling in my left thigh half way between my hip and my knee. When I felt around, I noticed a lump, and was panicked immediately. I felt for sure I had a metastasis in my leg. After feeling sorry for myself for a few minutes, I collected myself, returned to mindfulness and thought rationally about it. I hadn't read that bladder cancer metastasizes to the soft tissue, but I was still worried. I called the hospital to leave a message for Dr. Halberg. I hardly slept the rest of the night.

In the morning, Dr. Halberg's office called to say that she was off for the day, but they moved my follow-up appointment from July 2 up to June 24, so I'll see her on Tuesday. In the meantime, my friend, Dr. Marty Rossman called about another matter and offered to look at the lump. I went to his office and he confirmed what I now suspected was a lipoma - a fatty tissue that is no threat to anything. I've had a rather large lipoma on my back for as long as I can remember, and I don't have a clue where it came from.

I was a basket case for the rest of the day! I couldn't work, and I could barely function. I had to take care of one of my daughters, and we met a few friends for lunch at Kitty's Place. This was the nicest part of my day.

## 06/21/97: Separate Cars, Separate Rows

This was one of the first days that I didn't think much about the cancer. I worked in the morning and early afternoon to catch up on some coding that I haven't been able to do because of feeling so bad. I also had lunch with the girls and made two copies of the graduation tape. Then I did a mind story and took a long bath. By the time I was done with these activities, I was ready for a night out on the town. We took our kids to the R. and J.'s house where we met M. and M. R. and their kids. All the kids stayed together and we went out for pizza and a movie. The men drove in one car and the ladies in another. We even sat in separate rows in the movie. We saw, "Ulee's Gold."

## 6/22/97: Another No-Cancer Day!

Today was another day that you wouldn't think I had cancer unless you asked! I spent the morning scanning images from the graduation and Father's day last week. In the afternoon, we went to visit friends in San Mateo, and we took a walk that was the longest walk I've been able to manage since completing the chemotherapy. I didn't think too much about my disease until I arrived home exhausted. Then I felt it in spades and choose to listen to Thich Nhat Hanh.

## 6/23/97: No Pot stickers for my Chop Sticks

Today I'm back to healing. I went to see G. T. this morning and spent about an hour teaching her how to do a mind story. Then I thought I was scheduled in for a Feldenkrais Functional Integration lesson, but it turned out to be an hour and a half massage, and was it wonderful. It took me a little by surprise to have the massage, but she did such a good job, I didn't mind! I remember crying several times, as she was working on my shoulders, and she said that she felt that all of the poisons are out of my system at last. We then had lunch together in the shopping center at a Chinese restaurant.

Next, I went to see Leslie Davenport. While I was waiting to see her, I managed to get a little work done. The session with her was so fine! I seem to come out of there with profound insights and a lot of wisdom. She really validated my use of mindfulness in my healing process. I am really fortunate to have three such remarkable healers in my life who I love very much. Of course I'm referring to Gail, Leslie, and Anna Halprin, who is getting a life-time achievement award for choreography at Duke University as I write. I'm grateful for my physicians, Drs. Neuwirth, Gullion, and Halberg, and I feel that they were wonderful technicians who implemented a protocol that I found in my own research. But I really feel that a lot of my physical healing and all of my mental and emotional healing has come through the hands of Gail, Leslie, and Anna.

### 6/24/97: Moxibustion

Today was another day of healing. I spent the morning working, but then went to see Marty Rossman at 1:15 for acupuncture and Dr. Halberg at 3:00 for a follow-up visit. The emotional impact of the acupuncture treatment was unsuspected. I have had acupuncture before, but today I really felt the presence of someone who I know loves me as well. He worked on the kidney meridian with needles for just a short time and then he applied moxibustion to the same meridians. Moxibustion is "the burning on the skin of the herb moxa." In these days, they have sticky ends that you place on the meridians. Marty gave me a week's supply so that I could apply the moxibustion to myself in between visits.

We had to wait an hour to see Dr. Halberg, but it was not so bad except for the fact that I had to reschedule my eye exam. She was her kind, caring self, in spite of being an hour behind schedule. I felt that she really paid attention to my physical and emotional needs, as I try to understand the effect healing on my life. She didn't think anything of the lump I discovered last Friday, and said that it should be watched. She outlined my program for continued treatment, which consists of a chest X-Ray, complete blood count and blood chemistry, and cystoscopy every three months for the first year, every four months for the second year and every six months for the third through sixth year. I feel comfortable with this schedule, and the first thing I have to do is get the X-Ray, probably Thursday.

In the evening, my wife and I attended our respective groups at the Center for Attitudinal Healing. I was very touched by the stories people told, and I guess that's why I keep coming back. I spoke mostly about how much love was coming into my life and how much difficulty my wife is having with being my primary care taker. The latter idea was picked up by some of the other members of the group. I really felt a lot of compassion for care givers. Remember, I was in that role when my son was sick 21 years ago!

### 6/25/97: Hi Ho, Hi Ho...

Today I went to work in Menlo Park. Many people expressed how glad they were to see me, and I felt very supported. Now I am going to start work on the next generation project and try to contribute as much as I can.

When I got home, I tried out the moxibustion on myself. It seemed to have some effect, but I was too exhausted from setting up the environment and the long time in the car to go to and from work.

### 6/26/97: What's All This Chemotion About?

This morning I went for a chest X-Ray, but I won't know the results until tomorrow. I'm a little concerned, but not nearly as much as I am about my emotional state. It keeps rising and falling, just like my breath in the belly!

Cancerport was a bit disappointing this morning. I thought I would be able to share more of the emotional content of my life, but there were so many people there that I didn't feel comfortable letting it all hang out. Many people complained of care that was not so good and one person said that she had to take charge herself. I realized that she was right and that this was what I had been doing and need to keep doing.

Chemotion is a term I just created. It refers to the emotional ups and downs that have been occurring in me over the past three weeks, since the completion of my chemotherapy. I like the word, and I'm going to continue to use it. I went to speak with D. S. about chemotion. She has been living with ovarian cancer since 1991, and has been sending my get-well cards almost weekly. She is a person with a high level of self-esteem and a strong will to live. She shared with me her similar experiences with swinging emotions, and I felt quite comforted.

### 6/27/97: Master Ma

This morning, I had my eyes examined because I broke my frames. I found out that the insurance plan only pays for frames every other year, so I would only be covered for the exam and lenses. I opted to take the frames to the place I bought them, since my prescription hardly changed. They sold me a new frame at a replacement price (basically half of retail) and put the lenses in right on the spot!

After the exam, I went to Marin General Hospital for a Qi Gong lesson with Master Ma. He is Chinese and has been in this country only seven years. Even though his English was broken, I was able to understand what he said. He taught us the basic posture and the basic energy movement exercise. These were fairly simple and somewhat close to what my friend had taught me. Then he had us sit down and do an energy channeling exercise through our lung tips visualizing white light coming through our thumb and small finger joined together and placed over the opposite lung tip. Thus our arms were crossed, our backs straight and knees shoulder distance apart.

One of my neighbors died yesterday of metastatic prostate cancer. Although I didn't know the man at all, his wife was always kind. I really felt sad about his death and for the children he left behind.

### 6/28/97: Spectacular Fireworks!

I played one set of doubles the morning and it felt like I had played for three hours after the first time I served. I'm definitely not back to normal, but can you imagine the joy I felt, just hitting the ball after such a long time?

Someone gave Marty Rossman tickets to the A's game, so we took the girls to the Oakland Coliseum to see the A's lose 2-0 on two homers by the same guy. The game was followed by the best fireworks display I'd ever seen! It was so much fun! I felt fine, even though I did play tennis in the morning.

### 6/29/97: Naughty Marietta

My son had a leading role in Victor Herbert's Naughty Marietta in the San Jose Lyric Theater production today at the Montgomery Theatre in downtown San Jose. He played the part of the villain, Etienne Grandet. His performance was marvelous. His voice was the clearest and most understandable of any of the leading singers. Especially because he is a very nice person, he was a convincing villain.

### 6/30/97: Anna's Back!

I phoned the radiation oncology department to find out the results of my X-Ray from last Thursday. The person who answered the phone said that the results were wonderful! I had her repeat the statement three times just to be sure I got it!

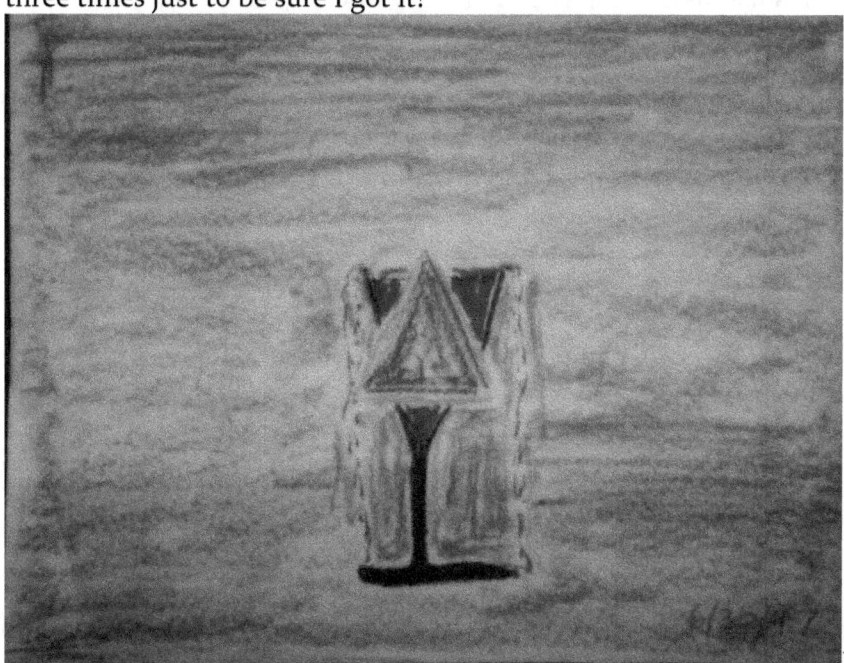

I went to G. T.'s Feldenkrais class in Tiburon this morning and then followed her to her office for a Functional Integration (FI) lesson. The class consisted of standing and kneeling lessons that served to loosen up my neck and shoulders. It was more strenuous than any of the previous lessons because we were standing most of the time. The FI session was wonderful! Her healing hands and gentle manipulations of my body made me fully relaxed.

In the evening, I went to Anna's class. She shared her experience at the American Dance Festival, and I was exceedingly happy for her triumph! She sparkled with light as she talked about the performances that she led, and she said that the response was phenomenal!

In the class, we did movements that were so similar to the Feldenkrais lesson that it made me realize the beauty of both techniques. Anna incorporated some movements that were familiar to me from doing the "Strengthening Your Immune System through Mind and Movement" exercises described elsewhere. As tired as I was from a full day of activities, I found the movements we did very invigorating and energy producing. Towards the end of the movement segment, Anna had us develop the theme of gathering, lifting, and sending away. Many of the participants drew pictures of their experience of gathering, lifting, and sending away. My drawing was of the goblet that I had visualized in a guided imagery session with Leslie Davenport. It represents my heart overflowing with love and vital energy. The inverted triangle represents a tap into the universal source of infinite love and vitality.

### 7/1/97: Another Busy Day

I began my day by trying to solve a problem at work, and I've been at it almost all day, except for my consultation with Michael Broffman and my acupuncture session with Marty Rossman.

The meeting with Michael Broffman produced some unexpected results. In the first place, what my wife has been saying about my diet is true. Michael told me to eat a low fat, high fiber diet, which eliminates many of my favorite foods, such as prawns and muscles. He is going to provide me with details about what I should avoid and what I should eat. Secondly, I had the startling realization that I'm not through with my disease. I still have a long way to go and the test procedures are not fun! I felt depressed from these two realizations, and I have been having difficulty dealing with them.

Since my wife took my appointment with Leslie Davenport, I took the opportunity to take a walk in the Cascade region of Mill Valley. The path leads to a waterfall, which is very nice, even now that it is not gushing with water. I spent about forty-five minutes there, practicing mindfulness and listening to the sound of the waterfall.

During my acupuncture treatment, I felt a burst of energy, and this gave me enough energy to continue working on the bug I'm trying to fix. Now I'm exhausted, but I continue to push on.

In the evening, my wife and I went to the Center for Attitudinal Healing for our respective groups. I spoke about my diet changes and feelings about not being finished with my disease. I also spoke about my wife's difficulties. The group was really supportive in an unusual way this evening.

### 7/2/97: An Incredible Transformation

Even though I felt better after the group last night, I woke up feeling terrible again. The feelings were mostly about diet and that I still had a long way to go with my illness. I was turned into myself when I showed up for a massage with G. T.. For me, this woman is the most remarkable healer. After about thirty minutes, I felt my heart starting to open again, and the pain and suffering over diet and disease seemed to lessen to such an extent that I was finally present again. I could, once again, bring my awareness to my breathing and re-establish mindfulness. It was one of the most remarkable transformations I've made in my whole healing process! I left her office feeling really great.

This was topped off by an extremely exciting session with Leslie Davenport. I spoke about the diet and disease feelings a little, but they had lost their sting. I began to focus on getting guidance on how to develop the workshop on "Zen and the ART of healing" with G. T.. I began to see old images from the seventies coming back this time with a specific goal in mind, and in the end, Leslie invited Gail and I to practice teach in her Wednesday class on July 26!

### 7/3/97: Hakone Gardens

After spending many hours on Monday, Tuesday and Wednesday on fixing the bug I'm working on, I felt a need for some time away from the computer. My sister in Redwood City agreed to take the kids today, so my wife and I spent time in Los Gatos, Saratoga, and especially Hakone Gardens. The weather was extremely hot in that part of the Bay Area and it really zapped my energy. We wound up visiting our friends in San Mateo and staying there until my sister brought the kids.

### 7/6/97: The Long Weekend!

I haven't written much about the long weekend, because not much is happening. I spent most of the fourth just hanging out. On the fifth, we took my daughter to visit a friend in Alameda and then visited my cousins in Berkeley. By three o'clock, I was exhausted and we came home. Today, I felt a little better and got out for a morning walk and a little tennis in the afternoon. I came home exhausted, but not as bad as yesterday. Now I'm catching up on some work.

### 7/7/97: Moon Set Over Corte Madera Creek

I was invited to play tennis with some of my favorite players this morning, but by ten o'clock, one person did not show up and the other person left without checking out the situation. I was rallying with the fourth person and someone he had found to hit with until the whole group was there. But just rallying like that is still too strenuous for me, and so I decided to attend the Feldenkrais class in Tiburon. This turned out to be a good choice because my back and knees were starting to hurt and the Feldenkrais lesson helped remove the tension.

In afternoon, I went to a session with Leslie Davenport. I had been feeling jittery all day for unknown reasons, and Leslie helped me relieve the tension. In the guided imagery, I felt myself return to mindfulness and I experienced a great sense of peace as I left her office.

Since it was too late to go home for dinner and get back to Marin General for Anna Halprin's class I invited B. F. to meet me at Pacific Cafe for dinner. After dinner, we went to the class taught by Liz Damtsey and Julie Emden. The focus of the class was different from all of the other classes, but it was definitely a refreshing change. We spent about thirty minutes talking about the pros and cons of body work in the context of our class situation, and finally, after a demonstration by out two leaders, we all agreed to give it a try. It turned out to be magnificent! I partnered with B. F., and we really connected quite well.

The massage began on the occipital part of the neck where the neck meets the head. We moved from there to massaging the scalp. Next, we placed our palms over the eyes of our partner and began massaging the face, cheeks and jaws. Next we placed our hand on the top of the chest, and just left them there for a few moments. From there, we moved to one shoulder, which we simply raised and lowered at the scapula. Then we worked on the arm by stretching it, and moving the joints of the wrists, elbows, and shoulders. After doing the other shoulder and arm, we began working on one of the legs. First we pulled the leg gently, and rotated it in the hip socket. Then we moved the foot to a standing position near the other knee. We lifted the leg at the knee and gently moved it towards the chest. After testing just how far we could go, we pressed on. Next we rotated the leg at the knee to loosen up the hip joint. We finished with the first leg by massaging the feet and then stroking the entire leg. After doing the same procedure on the second leg, we ended the session by placing our palms on the soles of the feet.

I felt that it was equally good to give as to receive. I enjoyed working with B. F., because she was really loose and trusting. This inspired me to be loose and trusting also.

We then did a quick drawing of whatever images came to us during the massage. I drew a picture of one person giving a massage to another in such a way that the giver and receiver couldn't be distinguished. They had merged and become one in the process. At this point, it is a bare sketch, and would not photograph to well for this page.

### 7/10/97: Getting Back to Normal

On Tuesday, I had an excellent acupuncture session with Dr. Rossman. He said that he felt my qi starting to flow like never before. I was encouraged by his remarks.

I spent the day on Wednesday at work. I'm starting to get a lot of pressure to complete certain tasks, so I've been working a lot lately.

Thankfully, I had a session with Leslie Davenport today, squeezed in between my work schedule. She is truly wonderful! She always helps me return to center!

### 7/11/97: Upsetting the Apple Cart

Once again, I felt a lot of pressure from work this morning, and I started about 5:15 A. M. I felt okay with this, as I anticipated a massage from G. T.. My wife had it in her mind that I should cancel my massage and spend time with my daughter. She went off for the day and was so attached to this idea that she gave me no peace. No matter what, the massage was wonderful! Gail is so kind and understanding that she helped to relieve all of the tension I felt from my wife. She even gave me good advice on how to behave with her when she got home from the wine country.

Because of earlier problems, I did not go to the opening session of Psyhchotronic Healing with Patricia Frisch, Ph. D., and Ruth Scott, both long time students of Nicholi Levashov and psychic healers. Instead, my wife and I went to visit Dr. Gerald Freedman (no relation!), a friend from the Center For Attitudinal Healing who lost his beloved last Monday. We brought candles and were really very touched by the atmosphere in his house and the other visitors. The candle light added a feeling of holiness to an already sensitive environment. Gerald has written many beautiful poems and haiku in connection with his wife's illness, and has given me permission to publish them on the web site.

### 7/12/97: Psychotronic Healing

Having made my peace with my wife the night before, I felt comfortable attending Patricia's workshop. Patricia and Ruth seemed to capture the essence of Nicholi's teachings. Although I missed the introduction the night before, I think I fit in nicely with the energy of the group. During the early morning sharing, I spoke about my cancer and my healing. I was especially interested in Nicholi's model of infection, which incorporates genetic and environmental causes, as well as in-utero effects. I think that there is real value in this psychotronic healing, and I've been trying it out with some friends at a distance.

During the lunch break, I had a remarkable time! I walked up to Union Street and had lunch in an Italian restaurant. My table was on the side walk, and I took delight in watching all the shoppers and passerby.

### 7/13/97: Marin Feels Healing Energy

Today was full of excitement! I began the day with two sets of doubles, which I managed to play with a remarkable degree of competence. There followed an hour bath and a brief nap. When I awoke, I had some lunch. Then I began writing and called Gerald Freedman to ask his permission to publish his poems and haiku on the web. To my surprise, he told me that I was famous! The article I had sent to the Marin Independent Journal on Monday appeared almost entirely in an article entitled, "Marin feels healing energy" on the front page of the "Lifestyles" section. I was extremely delighted to hear this news. A copy of the original paper that I submitted is on this web site as http://yellowsteam.org/healers.htm. The editor left out some information about Feldenkrais with G. T. and all that I said about Nicholi Levashov, but quoted most of the rest of the article. I imagine they left out Nicholi because he is from San Francisco.

In my excitement, I phoned Anna Halprin, G. T., Barbara Rose Billings, and Michael Broffman. Marty Rossman is on his way to Oregon with my daughter, so I'll tell him about it when I next speak with my daughter.

### 7/14/97: Planning the Workshop

G. T. and I met today to plan or workshop on "Mindfulness and ART in Healing." We are doing a practice teaching next Wednesday. Trying to cut a two day workshop into two hours is a bit difficult!

I didn't make it to Anna Halprin's class tonight, but I had a good time with my daughter. We went for a bike ride and then out to dinner.

## 7/15/97: The Healer's Healer

I had four remarkable experiences today! The first was sending off my wife and my younger daughter for a day by themselves, and they didn't know where they were going or when they would be back. It turns out that they spent the night in Gualala, on the Pacific Coast.

The second thing that happened gave me the most pleasure! I went to see G. T. for a Feldenkrais lesson. She began working on me and paused a few times without explanation. I asked her what was wrong, and found out that her right shoulder was hurting her and she had difficulty working. I asked her to trade places and proceeded to do a "zero balancing" treatment on her. I spent quite a bit of time with the treatment, and she was healed to the extent that she could continue working the rest of the day without a problem.

The third thing occurred during my visit to Dr. Gullion. I think he felt a little hurt that I didn't include him in my list of healers in the article, but I explained that I was just writing about "alternative" healers. So maybe I ought to write a letter to the editor to explain my lack of mention of the physicians that supported me during the Shipley protocol. He also mentioned that I was doing very well and didn't need to come back for three months!

Finally, I felt very sad at the Center for Attitudinal Healing because we lost another member. It was someone I liked a lot, and was just getting to know. Several other people were experiencing great difficulties. It was such a heavy night that the good news that I had to share lacked the spark that I wanted to offer to help healing. However, many people were very pleased with the article.

## 7/16/97: A Slow, Slow Day

After all the excitement of the past few days, I was bound to come to a screeching halt, and today was it! I could barely focus on work, and needed to nap shortly after lunch! Then, one of the members of my Conscious Evolution circle called me to go for a walk in Blythedale Canyon. I accepted without hesitation, and we had a nice walk together under the canopy of redwoods.

## 7/17/97: Renewing Friendship

Today I went to work, but I took a long lunch with V. R., one of the members of my small enneagram circle. We spoke about our lives in an open and touching way, as we usually do in our group. She and I have been friends for six years now and I really care for her and what wisdom she is able to speak.

## 7/20/97: Cultivating Family Value

The past few days have been filled with work, tennis, and cultivating family values. I played tennis on Friday and had my session with G. T. canceled, so I continued to work on Sniffer bugs. Yesterday, I managed a nice walk with my wife, in between work and going out to dinner. Today, in addition to playing tennis, I managed to fix the Sniffer bugs, and spent a lot of time preparing for the workshop on Wednesday.

## 7/21/97: Rehearsal

I spent most of the day with G. T., as we had to rehearse our presentation of Mindfulness and ART in Healing for Wednesday. Our meeting was full of joy and excitement, because we felt so good about what we were planning to do. Our long range plans include forming a non-profit corporation to apply for grants to present our workshop so that cancer patients aren't burdened with the additional expense of the workshop. We also spoke about how Gail's experience with various artistic media would fit naturally into the creative aspects of the workshop.

The workshop combines mindfulness as a healing practice with guided imagery, movement, and various forms of creative activity to encourage a powerful healing energy to evolve from within. More information about this workshop will be posted to our web site shortly. The agenda we decided on for the presentation on Wednesday includes the following:

1. Invocation to bind the group together
2. Check-in of all the participants
3. Guided mindfulness meditation
4. Opening to the breath exercises, maintaining mindfulness
5. A Feldenkrais awareness through movement segment done on chairs
6. If we have time, we'll have them produce some art work based on their experience of the day

7. Sharing
8. Closing

I'm getting really excited about this!

## 7/22/97: The End of a Phase

Today marks the end of a phase of my recovery. Tomorrow, I begin a new "career," which I have been looking forward to since my son got well. Finally, I have the courage and the opportunity to do something about educating people on how to make appropriate decisions for their medical care. There were times today that I found myself jumping up and down with excitement.

It was mostly an eventful day of work, as I solved a serious problem. In the evening, we went to the Center for Attitudinal Healing. It seems that a lot of people were jumping up and down this week! It was a wonderful meeting, and I was really happy to attend. I found myself really paying attention to the guidelines and principals, as if I never heard them before. Also, it was easy to listen to people's stories with compassion and understanding.

## 13 - MY NEW CAREER

### 7/23/97: Mindfulness and ART in Healing

Today was one of the best days of my life! G. T. and I led a two hour workshop in Leslie Davenport's wellness group at Marin General Hospital. The group was so pleasant and open to experiencing what we were there to give that the two hours just flew by as if they were only minutes. I took much pleasure in telling my story and leading the mindfulness meditation, and I was very impressed with Gail's handling of the check in and Feldenkrais lesson. The feedback was phenomenal! We are ready to take this concept around to healing centers everywhere!

This is our idea: We will set up a non-profit organization so that people who want to take our workshop can do so without financial burden. We will apply for grants and accept donations from wealthy people who have been helped by our cause. We will use this money to offer scholarships to those people who can't afford to pay for our services, and we will still draw our salaries from the corporation. The concept is still under development, and we are open to suggestions and contributions. Naturally, sales of *Healthy Cells Grow All By Themselves* will help promote our workshop, and our workshop will help promote sales of the book. Eventually, we will publish a book together based on the workshop. All it takes is time and money!

After the workshop we had lunch at an authentic Mexican restaurant and Gail gave me another one of her magnificent healing massages. Her work on my abdomen and bladder continue to inspire my complete recovery. I am very grateful for our relationship!

### 7/24/97: Insight Does It Again!

In my session with Leslie Davenport this morning, I was feeling a little down because of a series of bad dreams I had the night before. In two of the dreams, I was trying to escape. In the first one, I had to step through a lot of broken glass on the floor. I saw the broken glass and my shattered dreams from the past. During the session, I was able to reframe the broken dreams and create new ones. But, the second dream was more difficult to reframe. In this dream, I saw an opening in the prison fence and a car stuck in the railroad tracks. I managed to get in the car and drive it up the hill that was in front of the car, when I realized that the road had no exit out of the prison, so I was stuck. These two dreams brought out the seed so of doubt in me, and I was feeling a little desperate. In my session with Leslie, I was able to not only reframe the first dream, but I was able to see the joy that I was bringing to people, rather than the suffering, and I felt completely better. I took a walk along Corte Madera Creek, and felt the joy of insight.

## 7/27/97: Busy Days

I have been very busy the last three days with tennis, work, and family. However, the main thing has been getting the bugs out of the Sniffer! Now they are gone and I feel a little freed up.

My wife is off to Carmel for three days and I have the girls. This should be interesting!

## 7/28/97: Six Months Later

I spent most of the morning doing work and then went out to play tennis with my younger daughter. We had a nice lunch together and then her friend came over. Later in the day, I met G. T. for dinner and Anna Halprin's class. Tonight, Gail came for me, as my support person, but from now on, I think that she is going to come for herself! She had such a marvelous time.

In Anna's class, we did movements that reminded me of what Gail taught last Wednesday at our workshop. We began with massaging our feet, and then migrated to moving the rest of our bodies and especially our pelvises. As a result of earlier sharing, the theme of the evening was anger and determination. It was viewed that the energy of anger and the energy of determination were of the same nature. My drawing reflected my determination to get well. It began as an image of a boy jumping up and down, but since I didn't have the artistic skills to represent such an action, it turned into what looked like fireworks triggering other fireworks! Or, I even thought that it represented a one thousand petal lotus with each petal having one thousand petal lotuses upon it. It was a marvelous event!

## 7/29/97: Good Feedback!

G. T. and I had lunch with Leslie Davenport today to discuss her thoughts about our workshop last Wednesday. Her reaction was excitingly positive! She thought that the guided mindfulness meditation was wonderful, and she even wanted to use some of what I said in her guided imagery practice! As far as the Feldenkrais lesson was concerned, her only criticism was that Gail taught the lesson from a script, and it would have gone over better if she had memorized the movements. Gail accepted this comment with grace and charm, and the willingness to do so.

Since my wife was returning this evening, I wanted to make it somewhat special! I cleaned the house with the help of my daughter and bought her some roses. I even offered to make dinner for her, but she had had enough food over the past three days! It was nice to have her home again, and after apologizing profusely for all the mistakes I made, she seemed to settle into being home again.

### 7/30/97: Short Term Vision

In my session today with Leslie Davenport, I touched on several important areas. The first was trying to decide between a massage Friday morning or playing tennis. Thinking about the weeks ahead, it became clear that a massage would work better for me, even though I have finally been invited to become a regular in a foursome that I have been substituting in for the past two or three years! I see a lot of massages and a lot of tennis in my future!

My short term vision was that a lot of the issues I'm dealing with in regards to my illness will be cleared up in September, after I spend six days with Thich Nhat Hanh and have my cystoscopy exam the week after. Somehow, I sensed that there would be some clarity in my life about the issues around my illness as well as other aspects.

### 7/31/97: Nobody Wants to Go to Pleasanton!

I spent the whole day in Menlo Park. NGC just bought a company in Pleasanton, and it turns out that the group that I'm part of is the one group that has been chosen to work closely with the merged company! It was proposed that we all commute to Pleasanton, but this did not go over big with anyone except my boss, who lives there. I don't think my live would change much, since I'm a telecommuter, but it radically affected some of the other people in the group. Fortunately, NGC is open enough to reconsider its decision!

### 8/1/97: A Great Massage!

Today, I had a wonderful massage from G. T.! It was a hard decision to make - between tennis and massage, but in the end, the massage won out! I had such a good time!

## 8/10/97: Ten Days Later

It's been over a week since I've had an opportunity to write in these pages. Two weekends have gone by, and a week of hectic activity. I've finally become a "regular" for tennis with D. F. and E. M. on Mondays and Fridays. I've been a substitute for years and now I'm finally playing all the time. This changes a couple of things around for me. It means that I will have to miss G. T.'s Feldenkrais lessons at D. B.'s house. It also ties up two mornings a week, but it's what I want to do.

Last week I went to Anna Halprin's class on Monday, which was led by Julie. We performed a "hands" ritual, and my drawing was of hands in various positions. They were all variations of "loving hands", even though none of the drawings had that name. They were called, "praying hands", "begging hands", "healing hands", and "just hands". The "begging hands" came from an insight I had while doing the ritual: we are all beggars, asking for just one more day on the earth, but there is no one to beg, and no one to answer. Therefore praying and begging amount to the same thing. We need to take responsibility for our own lives and allow other people to live around us.

I had a great Feldenkrais lesson with Gail on Tuesday and a wonderful session with Leslie Davenport on Thursday.

Wednesday was quite exciting! I received calls from two publishers and met with a third. The first one wanted a copy of the complete manuscript for *Healthy Cells Grow All By Themselves*! I have been very busy converting the web pages to a document in the format required by this publisher. This has taken all of the time I usually spend writing the web pages.

The second publisher wanted to see a business plan for the book, which contains a synopsis and Table of Contents.

The third was Burton Goldberg, publisher of Alternative Medicine Digest and co-author of An Alternative Medicine Definitive Guide to Cancer. I told him my story and listened to his. Apparently, there is a lot more to the cancer cure than I or anyone one that I know is currently aware of and Goldberg's book has many new answers. I don't quite know where this relationship is going, but it could be very interesting. He especially likes my ideas of teaching people about cancer alternatives, through Mindfulness and ART in Healing. He thought that my idea to form a non-profit corporation to raise money to offer the workshop for free to financially handicapped patients was quite viable.

### 8/15/97: A Family Vacation

Today, we celebrated my younger daughter's birthday in Santa Barbara. We drove down here yesterday, only to find out that the reservations that had been confirmed were purged from the computer of the Pacifica Suites. Fortunately, someone canceled in time and we were able to get in.

I was especially exhausted today, for reasons unknown. The days before the trip were pretty much normal for me. I had a massage on Tuesday, but had to leave immediately for a meeting in Menlo Park. Wednesday, my wife and I had a joint session with Leslie Davenport. The session was fairly stressful, as many difficulties came up, but I seemed to recover from that session pretty well. So basically, I don't understand why I was so exhausted today.

### 8/19/97: Another Birthday Celebration!

Today, we took five eighth graders to Windsor Water Works in honor of my daughter's birthday, and wouldn't you know it, there was rain in August in Northern California! We were there long enough to enjoy the slides, however.

The rest of the Santa Barbara trip was about the same for me. I didn't recover my energy until today. I didn't sleep well, in spite of comfortable accommodations. The kids enjoyed the shopping mall, and I really felt closer to my wife. She was very caring and supportive of me during the trip. We had a really nice dinner together on Saturday night, leaving the kids in the room with more than enough pizza and Chinese chicken salad.

### 8/22/97: Feldenkrais with Harold

On Wednesday, I had another session with Leslie Davenport, and today, I met with her with my wife for the second time. Things went much better this time, and we seemed to get along better after the session. I was careful to express what I thought would work for me and

I felt that Mala really got it.

Earlier, I had a Feldenkrais lesson with Harold at the Feldenkrais training led by Anat Baniel. Although the session was not as good as I am used to, it worked well for me. Harold runs several old folks homes and his daughter runs physical therapy studios in the Chicago area. Gail and I took Harold out for lunch to tell him about our workshops. His reaction was favorable and he said that he would talk things over with his daughter and get back to us. His story about his illness and how he came to the Feldenkrais training was fascinating, but I won't go into it here.

## 8/25/97: Anat Meets Anna

I brought Anat Baniel, G. T., and Nancy Aberle, a Feldenkrais practitioner in Santa Barbara to Anna Halprin's class this evening. The interaction among these wonderful teachers was wonderful. One of the members arrived at the class and was actually too sick to do anything. She wanted to be taken to the emergency room to see if there was anything they could do for her. She left with the lady that brought her and another member of our group.

This put the group in a rather somber mood, so Anna had us do a remarkable ceremony with Native American overtones. The movement brought us quite close together and we all felt better for ourselves and for the sick lady. It turned out that she was able to go home that evening.

## 8/28/97: Gabrielle Roth

This evening, I attended an evening with Gabrielle Roth, and American Shaman. Back in 1975 and 1976, I spent much of my time with Gabrielle, as her student and assistant. Her main contribution to my life at that time was to support me through the worst of my son's bout with cancer. In addition, I learned a lot about movement from her. She actually had trained with Anna Halprin. On the day my son went into the hospital for surgery of his tumor, I was supposed to go to Eselan with Gabrielle to assist her in her workshop. However, this was not to be. A month earlier, Gabrielle and I put on an amazing event to honor Rajneesh. We had about 250 people attend, and it was wonderful.

This evening was very nice for me. As Gabrielle entered the

auditorium, I greeted her and she remembered me by name. She had just recently told someone about my son's miraculous recovery 21 years ago.

After about thirty minutes of movement, Gabrielle began to speak about trialectics (although she didn't mention the name). From my understanding, trialectics teaches that for every active force and its corresponding passive force, there is a neutralizing force to go along with them. Gabrielle spoke about awareness, attention, and action in the context of ourselves, our one-on-one relationships, and our relationships to a group. These last three concepts fit nicely into the three instincts of the enneagram. In respect to awareness, attention, and action, Gabrielle spoke about thoughts, feelings, and bodily sensations - the three centers of intelligence. At an appropriate time in the discussion, I delivered a little speech about the advanced stages of these centers. I used my concept of playing tennis with mindfulness as an example of being about to move before you know how you will move, that is, very instinctually. The phenomenon occurs in athletes when they enter the "zone" of ultimate capability. This was an example of body awareness that goes beyond the normal range of effort. I similarly spoke about feeling things before you know what you will feel, giving rise to lucid dreams, clairvoyance, and other psychic phenomena. Finally, I spoke about having thoughts that seem to come out of nowhere in which you just simply know. With these capabilities in place, one being to experience what it is like to be another. Gabrielle was pleased with what I had to say, and told the crowd that this was the essence of what she was teaching.

By the way, earlier that day I had a wonderful session with Leslie Davenport.

## 8/29/97: Feldenkrais Training

Today I was G. T.'s subject at the Feldenkrais training. She was a little nervous, as she was being carefully observed by one of her teachers. I could feel her anxiety, but I went along with her as well as I could.

## 14 - DAYS WITH THICH NHAT HANH

### 9/6/97: "Pain, Love, and Happiness"

On Labor Day, I drove down to the University of California at Santa Barbara with Nancy Aberle, G. T.'s friend from the Feldenkrais for a six day retreat with Thich Nhat Hanh. We made the trip in about six and one-half hours, and enjoyed getting to know one another. I imagine that she is a wonderful Feldenkrais teacher.

I was truly amazed at the turn out for the retreat, and how well organized it was for so many people. I was placed in a dorm with an 85 year old gentleman, J. G. from Laguna Beach. He was truly marvelous the whole six days. It was wonderful to see a wealthy old Jew be so taken by Thay (a nickname for Thich Nhat Hanh).

Our meals were taken in silence in large tents set up by the dorm. The food was strict vegetarian for the entire six days, and it was remarkably good. I think I might have even gained three or four pounds!

The days began with walking meditation with Thay to and along the beach that runs at the edge of the campus. With each step, there is one inhalation and one exhalation. Naturally, I used "healthy..., free..." the whole time. After about thirty minutes of walking, Thay would sit on a dune practicing sitting meditation for about twenty minutes, and we would all join him. Then we would walk back to the central part of the retreat in the same manner as we walked to the beach. On Wednesday, Thursday, and Friday, I walked and sat with three feet of Thay during the period of walking meditation.

After breakfast, there was always a dharma talk - a talk about the teaching of Buddha and the practical application of them in a life of engaged Buddhism. I was familiar with about ninety per cent of what he spoke about, but the look on his face, the excitement in his voice, and the presence of his being are well worth the time spent.

Following Thay's talk, one of the monks or nuns led us in mindful movements, which I later learned are related to qi gong. I was especially interested in them because of my workshop plans with G. T. on "Mindfulness and ART in Healing."

The schedule called for sitting meditation after the dharma talk, but it usually changed because of an extra-long talk or other events. When I sat, I noticed that I was not obsessing about next week's diagnostic tests - a biopsy of a mass in my thigh, and a cystoscopy. I found myself able to maintain a degree of mindfulness that kept me pretty much in tune with the present moment.

The afternoons were filled with special interest groups, dharma discussions, and supposedly a period of sitting meditation. I attended a special interest group on death and dying led by Joan Halifax, Ph. D. Joan is an ordained Zen teacher in the line of Thich Nhat Hanh, Seung Sahn, and Bernie Glassman Roshi. She is the founder of Upaya and resides in Santa Fe, New Mexico. The first time we met, she spoke about being with the dying person without trying to fix them. If they were open to teachings about mindfulness, we should speak with them; otherwise, we should just be there with our mindfulness engaged in "loving speech and deep listening." The next morning, I had a private interview with Joan. I wanted to discuss my practice as it related to healing the cancer that was in my body. I could tell that she was deeply moved by my story, and she had me tell it again to a small group of her special interest group in the afternoon.

Following the special interest groups, there were dharma discussions. The first day, we had a tea ceremony, which was lovely. The other days, we spoke about Thay's dharma talk, the "Five Mindfulness Trainings", and other topics which people brought up. I found myself speaking a lot and sharing my story with this group also. We seemed to get very close in a matter of hours. I expect to continue my friendship with several of the people I met in my dharma discussion group.

The schedule called for sitting meditation after the dharma discussion groups. One afternoon, the thirty-four monks and nuns that were traveling with Thay from Plum Village were invited to demonstrate some of the chanting they do in their practice. The chanting was so wonderful. It seemed as if they all had wonderful voices. Thay, himself, introduced us to many of the monks and nuns.

On that same afternoon, Nancy came to visit me. After the chanting, we took a walk on the beach and I talked her into staying for dinner. She did not stay for the evening program.

The evening programs were varied and wonderful. Monday night, Thay gave an introductory dharma talk. Tuesday night, Sister Chan Khong offered "Five Earth Touchings". The five earth touchings consisted of acknowledging our physical ancestry, and our spiritual ancestry, along with honoring the ancestors who made freedom possible in our corner of the world. The final two touchings were to people we love the most and people we love the least. I was moved to tears by most of this experience.

I spoke with Sister Chan Khong the next day before lunch about the "Five Earth Touchings". I also told her about my illness and how I used mindfulness as a healing tool. She shared with me two stories about people who also used mindfulness with their illnesses. I then told her about "healthy cells grow all by themselves," and she said, "With your wisdom and Thay's teachings, you are going to be fine."

On Wednesday evening, there was a presentation of the Five Mindfulness Trainings offered by several people in the Order of Interbeing. I found this quite helpful, as I planned to take them along with the three refuges of the Buddha, the Dharma (teachings), and the Sangha (group of people in the practice of the dharma). In other Buddhist traditions, the Five Mindfulness Trainings are known as the Five Precepts for lay people practicing Buddhist meditation. I am going to try to get permission to put the text of Thay's Five Mindfulness Trainings on this site, but for now, I'll simply summarize the intent of each one.

1. Respect for life - non-killing
2. Respect for property - non-stealing
3. Avoidance of sexual misconduct
4. Respect for others - loving speech and deep listening - telling the truth
5. Avoidance of intoxicants - drugs, alcohol, certain TV programs, etc.

I have been practicing most of these precepts already, and the formal presentation was quite interesting. I took all five mindfulness trainings on Saturday morning when they were offered by Thay.

On Thursday evening, Sister Chan Khong presented the "Three Prostrations". These involved our relationship to time, space, and the whole stream of life. Once again, I was deeply moved.

The last night consisted of questions from the sangha and answers from Thay. He responded spontaneously to many wonderful questions.

The whole retreat reminded me of Thay's description of the life of the Buddha in Old Path White Clouds. The walking meditations suggested Buddha's travels in what is now India and Nepal. He walked everywhere with a sangha of about 1500 bhikkhus and lay people. The silent meals reminded me of how the bhikkhus would beg for food in the villages and towns and return to the forest to eat their meals together.

## 9/9/97: Back to Earth

The return to normal life was not too disheartening. Sunday, I felt a little exhausted. I took my wife out for a nice lunch because I thought I was going to a concert in Saratoga with my son. I was too tired to make the trip, however. Monday was a normal day of tennis and work. But today was different. I had to have a needle biopsy of the mass in my left thigh. I discovered this lump on June 20, and have been watching ever since. Today was the day to do something about it. I don't know the results yet, but the procedure was not too painful, and I was able to work when I got home. Even now, the pain is not too bad.

## 9/10/97: The Day of Reckoning!

This morning, I had a powerful and healing massage from G. T. in preparation for my cystoscopy examination this afternoon. Gail was really on today with her energy work as well as her massage technique. I think she gets better with each treatment.

In spite of this, I faced the cystoscopy with great fear of the unknown, and my fears were merely based on wrong perceptions on what actually occurred. The nurse inserted a local anesthetic in my penis and ten minutes later, Dr. Neuwirth inserted the cystoscope. The cystoscope consisted of a light through which he could see into the bladder, and channels for flushing fluids through. The good news is that he did not see any visible cancer, but the wash had to be sent off to the lab for a cytology examination. We'll know the results by Monday.

## 9/12/97: More Waiting

I found out today that the biopsy sample had to be send to Stanford University for more tests. Apparently, the tests that they could run at Marin General Hospital were not conclusive, so they needed to consult the expert in the field, Dr. Richard Kempson. I found out about all of this by repeated calls to Dr. Head without hearing anything in return. So I picked up the phone and called Dr. Jacques, the pathologist at Marin General and he told me the news. He identified the mass as a stromal tumor, either from fat or the nerve sheath, but he wasn't certain if it was malignant or benign. So here we have to wait through the entire weekend or more for the results. By the way, I also phoned Dr. Kempson, but he had not received the sample yet.

My session with Leslie Davenport was helpful in dealing with all of this stuff. I think I'll be able to make it through the weekend because of the Day of Mindfulness with Thich Nhat Hanh tomorrow!

## 9/13/97: A Day of Mindfulness

My day with Thay was wonderful. It felt like a day of nirvana, as it seemed to be a continuation of the retreat last week. Again, Thay's teachings, the mindful movements, and the earth touchings moved me deeply. There were 2500 people at Spirit Rock!

## 9/17/97: Thay's Lecture

This evening, we went to Thich Nhat Hanh's lecture at the Berkeley Community Theater along with 3500 people attending the lecture. It was fortunate that I planned to attend this lecture because not all of the news I got today was good.

Dr. Gullion had the results of the cystoscopy and the needle biopsy earlier in the day. While Dr. Neuwirth saw no visible signs of cancer, the wash of my bladder revealed atypia cells and other carcinoma cells, which could indicate that there is some microscopic cancer in my bladder. However, Dr. Halberg and Dr. Huang both assured me that these cells could be a result of the radiation. As a result, I have to go in for a biopsy under anesthesia on October 3 to have my bladder checked out.

The results of the needle biopsy of my left thigh were inconclusive. The preliminary indication is that I have a schwannoma, which has to be surgically removed in order to accurately identify it. This means another set of doctors at UCSF, and perhaps a three night stay in the hospital there. I have to be able to walk on my leg before they'll let me out of the hospital.

I had an opportunity to talk all of this over with Leslie Davenport after seeing Dr. Gullilon. She was very helpful, but I had already seen that although these procedures are complicated and time consuming, neither one of them are extremely dangerous.

## 9/22/97: Eric Vormanns

Eric Vormanns is a West African energy healer residing in Belgium. He is in Marin until September 29, and I was referred to him by Leslie Davenport. My session with him left me quite sad. Even though he thought the cancer would eventually go away, he thought that I was not doing what I came to this life to do. He thought that I should be writing, teaching, and practicing in the areas of healing and spiritual growth. I felt sad because I knew that I lacked the courage to devote my life to these activities. Of course, this web site and other activities contribute, but I don't feel that it is enough. I need to get Healthy Cells Grow All By Themselves published and appear on talk shows all over.

In the evening, I went to Anna Halprin's class. The picture I drew was quite amazing. It was called, "grib-it," and featured a frog and the stream of life. I felt quite good expressing myself through this drawing. It seemed to contain everything that I experienced in being with Thich Nhat Hanh.

### 9/24/97: CT Scan

I had an appointment with Michael Broffman this morning to go over the results of the two biopsies. His opinion was that I should have the schwannoma excised, primarily because it was on the bladder meridian. He didn't see any danger. He is waiting for the results the cystoscopy under anesthesia next week in order to change my protocol of vitamins and other supplements. My wife and I continue to be impressed with his vast knowledge of medicine, in general, and especially cancer!

In preparation for the surgery next week, I had to have a CT scan today. The only difficult thing about this procedure is that I had to drink more than a quart of barium sulfate in order to get a good contrast on the films.

### 9/25/97: Another Visit to the Doctor!

Again, in preparation for the surgery next Friday, I had to have another physical at Dr. Belknap's office. Fortunately, the blood work and the CT scan indicated no mets (metastases)! Thank Buddha for that!

By the way, all through these adventures since returning from Santa Barbara, I have been having wonderful sessions with Leslie Davenport and G. T.. I haven't reported much about them because they have had only a positive influence on my recovery. I have also been playing tennis, as usual.

## 10/1/97: A Confusing Day with Surgeons

When I first spoke with Dr. Gullion about the schwannoma, he referred me to Dr. Warren, a doctor at UCSF to do the surgery. On Monday, his office called me to say that Dr. Warren was going to be out of town for the next few weeks and recommended that I see Dr. Norton. Well, in tune with my attitude about doing the best possible research, I didn't want to see Dr. Norton without checking into the matter more fully. So, I asked Dr. Gullion what he thought, and he wanted me to speak with Dr. Warren first. Dr. Gullion finally called me back this morning at 11:00, while my appointment with Dr. Norton was at 10:45. I also had an appointment with Dr. Warren, so I missed both of them through all of the confusion. The point of all of this is that I want to be very careful about who keeps me from playing tennis for any period of time due to the surgery on my leg.

I finally took some time away with my wife over the weekend. After seeing Leslie Davenport on Friday, we took off to Gualala, a small town on the Mendocino coast. We spent two nights in different motels, each equipped with a Jacuzzi in the room. We had a wonderful time. The beach at Gualala is beautiful and awe inspiring.

## 10/8/97: An Unhappy Birthday to Me!

Today I turned 58, but what a miserable day it was. As you may know, last Friday I had my cystoscopy and biopsy under anesthesia at Marin General Hospital. The results were not favorable, but also not so bad. There was some microscopic cancer still on the bladder wall, but Dr. Neuwirth thought that it could be removed with one or two six week treatments of BCG. The cancer was down to grade I or II, so, all in all, it is slowly going out of my system. The BCG treatments start next Wednesday.

This morning, we went to the University of California at San Francisco (UCSF) to meet with Dr. Norton about the schwannoma. I expected a forty-five minute visit followed by a nice lunch at the Cliff House and a stroll through the de Young Museum or the Palace of the Legion of Honor. This would have been a lovely way to spend my 58th birthday, but Dr. Norton changed all my plans. He wanted to remove the schwannoma on Friday - the day after tomorrow! Dr. Gullion supported his plan, and it seemed reasonable based on getting that thing out of my leg before the BCG treatments begin. I was in a state of shock about the urgency in his analysis of my problems. He went so far as to say that the lipoma on my left shoulder blade should also come out. So I spent the rest of the day registering for the surgery on Friday.

I was a bit disappointed because I had worked so hard to get appointments with neurosurgeons next Monday. I thought that because the schwannoma was a nerve sheath tumor, it should be removed by a neurosurgeon. Dr. Gullion did not share my ideas about the neurosurgeon. He thought that Dr. Norton was better because he understood the oncology. Dr. Norton has done many of these, so I feel confident in him, but the schwannoma will be gone before I have a chance to see the other surgeons.

## 15 - ADDITIONAL TREATMENTS

### 10/18/97: Catching Up

Here I sit, ten days after my last entry, recuperating from two successive weeks of surgery. Last Friday I spent two nights in the hospital at the University of California in San Francisco (UCSF), one of the best teaching hospitals in the country. The surgery occurred on Friday, October 10 and lasted about two and one-half hours. I was in the recovery room for about three hours. The surgeon, Dr. Norton, excised both the schwannoma in my leg and the lipoma in my shoulder blade, both on the left side. The stay in the hospital was made much less unpleasant by the kind and courteous staff, and, in spite of much pain, I remained comfortable. At one time, last Saturday, there were ten visitors at once!

Getting up the stairs on Sunday morning was no picnic. I had to sit on each stair and push myself up to the next one with my good leg. I couldn't use crutches because of the lipoma incision. I've spent practically all of the last week lying in bed, doing mindful breathing, reading, and trying to get some work done. There was a lot of excitement this week, as Network General and McAfee are merging, and I missed all of the parties and announcements. On Thursday, I finally went out to see Dr. Norton, and yesterday I managed one half-hour sitting by the water in Sausalito. Dr. Norton said that the preliminary report on both biopsies was that they were benign.

I've had a mild case of post-operative depression, as I feel much like an invalid, having to use a walker or crutches to get around. Everything is starting to move forward now, however, and I expect to take part in some social activities this weekend. Wednesday, I see Dr. Norton and perhaps have the first of a series of BCG treatments in my bladder.

### 1/25/98: One Year Later

Two days ago, I received a call from Dr. Neuwirth's office that my cystoscopy from January 14 was negative! This means that there is no longer any cancer in my bladder, and I am well on my way to a complete recovery. It also means that I am in remission. What events led up to this wonderful result? I shall try to trace what happened since my last entry Father's day.

The summer was difficult to manage because of the effects of the chemotherapy. To help myself out, I continued body work, movement, therapy, and tennis. I did as much work as I could and was able to keep up with my assignments. I played tennis about twice a week, and that was all I could manage.

In August, we took a family trip to Santa Barbara in honor of my youngest's birthday. The trip was pleasant, but I was not recovered from the chemo. This, I was terribly exhausted most of the day and took restoril to sleep at night. My wife and I got along quite wonderfully, considering the three girls in the other room, and my inability to function most of the day.

September began with a wonderful experience at a meditation retreat with Thich Nhat Hanh in Santa Barbara. In a way, the retreat helped to prepare me for what was the beginning of extremely hard times. On September 9, I had a needle biopsy of the growth in my left thigh, and on September 10, I underwent a cystoscopy exam by Dr. Neuwirth. The needle biopsy was so unusual that the specimen was sent off to Stanford University. The result was that I have a schwannoma in my thigh, and the recommendation was to remove it.

Even though Dr. Neuwirth did not see any visible cancer, the washings had to be sent off to the lab for biopsy. Unfortunately, the result came back that I still had some dysplasia and carcinoma-in-situ. This result was extremely depressing to me, as I had counted on a clean result. Dr. Neuwirth, however, was not terribly discouraged, and he expressed confidence that a six week treatment of BCG would clear up any remaining cancer in my bladder.

On a positive note, my visit with Dr. Gullion and the accompanying blood tests were good. In addition, I had a CT scan on September 24, which revealed no sign of cancer elsewhere in my body. But these results didn't help avoid the pain and suffering that was to come.

On October 3, I went into Marin General Hospital for a biopsy under anesthesia to confirm the findings of the cystoscopy three weeks before. The results did indeed confirm that I still had carcinoma-in-situ and dysplasia, and that BCG treatments would be the recommended procedure.

Meanwhile, I made several appointments with various surgeons to discuss my schwannoma surgery, and on my 58th birthday, October 8, I met with Dr. Jeffrey Norton at UCSF. His arguments for immediate surgery were convincing and he said, "I can do it Friday!" In addition, he wanted to excise the lipoma under my left shoulder blade while he had me on the operating table. So, on Friday, October 10, I checked into the hospital. In the pre-op room, I pleaded one more time to make sure the surgery was absolutely necessary, but I was overruled. Dr. Norton did agree not to touch the lipoma if anything went wrong with the schwannoma.

Well, nothing went wrong, and both masses were excised. I spent the better part of three days in the hospital, and then I went home. Getting up the steps was quite a chore, which I managed by sitting on a pillow on each step. I had to get around the house in a walker for about a week, and then I could use crutches. The lipoma surgery prevented me from using crutches to get around after the surgery, and actually this is what kept me in the hospital for the extra days. You know how they want to get you out of the hospital as soon as possible these days.

I started physical therapy with Julie Wong at ProActive Physical Therapy in San Francisco on October 28. She was the same physical therapist that my wife used after her hip surgery last year. Julie is marvelous and highly recommended. I thoroughly enjoyed working with Julie. She taught me exercises to strengthen my shoulders and my legs, which I am still doing today, even though I am completely recovered from the two surgeries. All in all, I had six sessions with Julie.

I felt I was ready for the BCG treatments by October 29. Whereas the treatments themselves involve inserting the BCG directly into the bladder by means of a catheter, the precautions necessary when you get home are strenuous. Every time you urinate, you have to disinfect the toilet as well as yourself, because the bacteria are still active. I found this part to be quite annoying, and to keep this up for six weeks was a major undertaking. Furthermore, after the instillation, you must try not to urinate for at least two hours afterwards, so you have to stop drinking all liquids at least four hours before the treatment. What a hassle, but it beats the alternative hands down.

During this whole period, I felt quite depressed, and sought the help of Leslie Davenport, sometimes twice a week. Her help and guidance made the impossible just difficult, and I managed to pull through the whole thing. In addition, I managed to attend Anna Halprin's class as soon as I was able to get around. These two women have really helped me a lot throughout the entire duration of my illness.

On January 14, I had another cystoscopy with Dr. Neuwirth. The purpose of this procedure was to check on the effectiveness of the BCG treatments. Dr. Neuwirth made two statements that gave me hope that the treatments actually worked. He said that my bladder looked like one that had been treated with BCG, and that he could tell that I was taking high doses of vitamins.

Nine days later, I had the results. I had no cancer in my bladder! I had no dysplasia or carcinoma-in-situ! I was in remission! What a marvelous and wonderful ending to a very difficult year. Just two days before the one year anniversary of my gross hematuria, I found out that I no longer had cancer in my bladder.

### 2/5/98: HealthyWay Award!

Less than two weeks later, I received the following email from HealthyWay:

Dear Web Colleague,
Congratulations! Your site has won a HealthyWay Best of the Web Award!
After reviewing thousands of Web sites, the HealthyWay team has designated your site, "Yellow Stream -- A Bladder Cancer Diary", as one of the best online resources for health and wellness information.
A review and link to your site is provided from the Health Links section of HealthyWay. (http://www1.sympatico.ca/Contents/Health/REV_HTML/S21366.html) This section features links to over 10,000 Web sites, articles, and FAQs: Conditions & Diseases, Visit the Specialist, Disabilities, Alternative Medicine, Family Living and more. Only the very best of these sites are reviewed and rated by the HealthyWay team -- and "Yellow Stream -- A Bladder Cancer Diary" is among this select group.
As a result of its usefulness and quality as an online resource, we are pleased to announce that your site is a recipient of our Best of the Web Award.
ABOUT HEALTHYWAY:
HealthyWay is an award-winning Web site dedicated to helping people get well and stay well. The HealthyWay provides a balanced health focus, combining the elements of traditional medicine, complementary medicine, and healthy, active living. We've built online

health communities that overcome the limitations of time, distance, rarity of condition, and physical disabilities. Comprehensive, well organized resources plus a unique review/rating system helps people quickly and easily access relevant information and services.

ABOUT YOUR BEST OF HEALTH AWARD:

To collect your award, please visit the HealthyWay Winners' Circle http://healthcentral.sympatico.ca/awards/cgi-bin/HealthAward.pl?S21366, which contains instructions on how you can display the HealthyWay Best of the Web Award.

If you have any questions, please visit HealthyWay at http://healthyway.sympatico.ca/ or reply to this e-mail.

Best Regards,
Angela                                                           Warburton
HealthyWay
healthyway@sympatico.ca
http://healthyway.sympatico.ca/

---------------------------------------------------

If you are not responsible for adding our award icon and link to your site, please forward this to the appropriate person.

We apologize for the inconvenience. Thank you.

**2/22/98: Lessons Learned**

To continue my story, I'd like to share with you some of the lessons I've learned in dealing with cancer. First and foremost is the love and support of caring friends and family. For this, I am very thankful, and don't know exactly what to say beyond how difficult it would have been without them.

Secondly, I learned the value of doing my own research, and, at the same time, having the support of competent physicians and healers. I could not ignore the input of the doctors, but I knew enough to present a viable alternative. I am grateful to Doctors Harry Neuwirth, David Gullion, Francine Halberg, Sara Huang, Robert Belknap, Peter Carroll, Jeffrey Norton, Peter Klaphaak, and William Shipley for their willingness to put up with my radical approach to healing. When I think about the possibility of having had a radical cystectomy and compare it with the treatments I've had, I really count my blessing at having made the right decision for me. The radical cystectomy could have led to complications too numerous to understand at the time of the surgery. I am happy that I bypassed this option.

Thirdly, I don't have any clue about the direct effect of the cancer support groups, alternative medicine, supplements, body work, and psychotherapy had on the physical healing of my illness, but they were all indispensable for my emotional and mental healing. To this, I owe a debt of gratitude to Dr. Martin Rossman, Thich Nhat Hanh, Leslie Davenport, Anna Halprin, Michael Broffman, G. T., Elyse Genuth, Dr. Van Vu, Dr. Patricia Frisch, and Alan Sheets for their contribution to my healing efforts, be they of the body, emotions, mind, and spirit. I guess I'll never know whether these methods had anything to do with my healing, but I don't want to think about how it would be if I hadn't done them.

Finally, even with all the love and support of the people I've already mentioned, I have to acknowledge my own part in this process. I did my research, found a creative outlet for my experience in these pages, practiced mindfulness during critically ill times as well as healthy ones, and continued to look forward to a happy and healthy life beyond cancer. My goal has been to maintain as much mindfulness in all my activities as possible, including, but not limited to time on the tennis courts, walking meditation, computer work, and enjoyable outings with family and friends. My experience has been beneficial to other people, as well, through my web site, support groups and contact with friends taken ill by a similar disease. I am happy that I can help them, but not quite happy with the path that led me to the knowledge I have to do so.

In conclusion, let be state once again how important I think it is to combine the best of Western medicine with natural healing methods to come up with a treatment plan that can result in a cure. The process of healing the body must be accompanied by the process of healing the emotions, the mind and the spirit.

### 12/16/98: Another Year Has Passed

More than a year has passed since my last entry. I must say that 1998 was much better than 1997. I had cystoscopies in January, April, June, and November, and they were all normal - i. e., no cancer. I am now on a four month schedule for cystoscopies.

As far as the rest of my recovery is concerned, I continue to follow the directions of Michael Broffman as far as herbs, vitamins, and other supplements are concerned. I don't want to underestimate the effect of these supplements. I believe they are helping my body to cope with the foreign toxins that were introduced all of 1997.

I continue to play tennis and practice walking meditation. Once in a while, I got to Anna Halprin's class, but not as much as I'd like. I've dropped out of the other support groups I was attending. My family and friends continue to be my first line of support. It's pretty amazing that I've come out of this with such a clean skin!

## 3/26/00: Two Years Later

On January 19, 2000, I had a cystoscopy which resulted in atypical cells in the wash. However, I did not find out about this until several weeks later because I went to India on business and then to France for vacation. While in France, I went to Plum Village, where Thich Nhat Hanh (lovingly call Thay - beloved teacher) lives for most of the year. Plum Village consists of three hamlets: Upper Hamlet, where monks live; Lower Hamlet, where nuns live; and New Hamlet, also where nuns live and guests stay.

In India, I trained programmers at Cybermedia and visited the Osho Commune. This is a place where I had been in 1975! There were a lot of changes to the grounds of the ashram, but, even though Osho died, the atmosphere wasn't very different from 1975. My wife had been there as late as 1978. If you go there, you'll find lovely grounds and gardens, and workshops on just about any spiritual, psychological, or physical discipline you wish! I found it very much fun and enjoyed the food there so much.

Plum Village was another story. I arrived there during the Tet celebration of the Lunar New Year. The monks and nuns were immediately hospitable and welcomed me with open arms. The next several days were filled with feasting, consulting of the oracle, visiting the rooms of the monks and nuns, and talks by Thich Nhat Hanh. I found Plum Village to be one of the richest spiritual experiences of my life. I have such great respect for the sangha (community of monks and nuns) and this brought me even closer to Thich Nhat Hanh.

During one of the oracle readings, Thay spoke about how someone who thought they had cancer could be having a wrong perception and therefore talk themselves into the disease. After the session completed, I approached Thay with the question I had about my friend who was suffering with glioblastoma - the worst form of brain cancer. We took each other's hands and Thay said to me, "Perhaps you can consult the oracle!" Little did I know that the results of my cystoscopy were not negative.

A little while later, in the room of the abbess of Lower Hamlet, one of the senior monks answered the question for me. He said that the person should live her life as fully as possible in each moment. Five weeks after I returned home, my friend passed away. On the afternoon before her passing, she went out to lunch with her daughter. She fully lived up to the monk's response.

When I got home from my travels, my wife told me about the results of the cystoscopy. I went into a mild depression, knowing that I asked Thay about my friend, when, perhaps, I should have asked about myself! I wasn't ready to deal with a recurrence. Is anyone ever? On Wednesday, March 1, 2000, I went into the hospital for a biopsy under surgery, as recommended by Dr. Neuwirth. Two days later, I found out that all the tests were negative. I could breathe a sigh of relief!

## 11/26/03: Update through 2003

I am looking over the website today and correcting any broken links. I thought I would take this opportunity to record my progress over the past three years.

All of my children are home for Thanksgiving and it is wonderful to have everyone here. Micah lives in New York City and is doing quite well. Rachael lives in San Diego and is in her third year of college. She is studying architecture, which she has been talking about since she was seven!. Jessica is in Eugene, Oregon, where she studies journalism.

All of my health reports have been outstanding since the last entry. I had an MRI last April, but it was negative. Other than this, there hasn't even been a scare. Many consider that I have been cured.

In October, 2002, I was laid off from Network Associates. After my trip to India in 2000 (see above), I proceeded to train around three dozen Indian programmers in Dallas. Network Associates subsequently opened an R&D center in Bangalor and eliminated my job.

I almost immediately got a job at WildPackets, doing basically the same kind of work with network protocols. When Bush went into Iraq, WildPackets had many cancellations and so they cancelled my job. I've been working on packet analysis for NetPredict since September, 2000, but they are also struggling. I guess the most significant project I've been working on is the website for Jewels by Mala. The site is based on osCommerce, and I like the results. Please let me know what you think.

## 01/26/04: Seven Years Have Passed!

Seven years have passed since I presented at Marin General Hospital with blood in my urine. These have been interesting times in my life. My kids are now grown and off to college.

I was laid off from WildPackets in April, and haven't had a steady job since then. I've been working on several consulting projects and developing Jewels by Mala with my wife. The website is launched, but sales are slow.

Unfortunately, most of the information on this site is now 5-7 years old. I am considering doing more research in bladder cancer when I have the time, but this website should provide you with a guide to how to do the research yourself. We still think Michael Broffman has many good answers, and continue to direct people to

## 05/21/06: More than Nine Years Have Passed

Today, I begin revamping the web site by adding features that may improve the readability and access to information. I am also adding a section on books on cancer.

When I first started working on this web site, I only had done one site before The Enneagram in the Electronic Tradition. Now that I have developed Jewels By Mala, NewTerra, Jobs-Are-Us, Mountain Sangha, and MICAH Affiliates, as well as internal web sites for The Technical Committee, I have enough experience to do a better job on Yellow Stream.

In the meantime, I am experiencing excellent health. My last cystoscopy was in June, 2005 and everything was good. I am experiencing no after effects of the radiation or chemotherapy, other than ease of exhaustion.

My son, Micah is living in New York and doing computer graphics and web site development. He has started a theatre company, QED Productions with a group of his friends. He produced and acted in Tom Stoppard's Arcadia last November at the Greenwich Theatre, which Mala and I attended. The group plans three productions for next season. Come if you can!

Rachael is entering her last year in architecture school at Woodbury University in San Diego, CA. She is a lovely and kind young woman with a bright future.

Jessica graduates with honors and a double major in Spanish and Journalism from the University of Oregon in three weeks. She will be teaching in Spain in the fall under the auspices of the Spanish Consulate. Mazel Tov - Jessica.

Mala is a wonderful and supporting spouse. She is doing great work with her jewelry designs.

For the past four years, I have been intimately involved with the Mountain Sangha in Mill Valley. Our sangha practices in the tradition of Thich Nhat Hanh, whom I've written about in previous chapters. Please read *My Breakfast with Thay* to see what happened when I visited Plum Village for the second time in March, 2006. It was a wonderful visit!

My Buddhist practice now consists of morning meditation, tennis when possible, walking meditation, and reading of Buddhist scriptures. I am an aspirant in the Order of Interbeing. I am also working towards offering a class on *Mindfulness in Healing* through California Cancer Care and other institutions. The class is based on my experience, which is documented in these pages.

My tennis game continues to improve. I play for Harbor Point and our team went to the divisional playoffs last month as a wild card team. My partner and I won one match, but lost two others - one in a tie break. I try to play every day that I don't have to go to Palo Alto (where my office of TheTC [see below] is located).

I now have perhaps the best work in the computer industry. I am working as a consultant to the Technical Committee (TheTC) of the Department of Justice. TheTC is chartered to monitor the compliance of Microsoft with the antitrust settlement agreement which just has been extended until 2009. Because of the work I did between September, 2004 and December, 2004, 30 engineers have jobs and we are making sure that Microsoft correctly documents their proprietary networking protocols for licensees.

## 16 – A NEW EPISODE

### 4/21/10: The Brain Revealed: From Chemistry to Mystery

The Institute for Health and Healing (IHH) sponsored the Roberta E. Neustadter Mini-Medical series on The Brain Revealed: From Chemistry to Mystery. I attended the two previous evenings, so this was my third. The second talk was given Allison Shapiro, who made a remarkable recovery from a nearly fatal double stem stroke. I had met her about a year ago at a Saybrook event and we spoke for a long time.

The main highlight of Allison's talk was her paying attention to the slightest movement and making an effort to enhance the healing possibilities resulting from that attention. When our client heard this, she was very touched.

After the talks, I went to the rest room and noticed some dense fluid flowing more quickly than the rest. I knew it was time to call Dr. Neuwirth to schedule my annual cystoscopy. This actually also come coincidentally with my wife's urinary tract infection, which was treated with antibiotics.

### 4/28/10: Cystoscopy

As mentioned in the introduction, I had my annual checkup this day. It was actually six weeks past one year, but I was prepared to even wait longer to go in, due to twelve years of a clear bladder. For the first time, Dr. Neuwirth found two small polyps in my bladder. I was surprised when he removed the scope without taking samples for biopsy like he usually did. He told me to get dressed and he would come back and talk to me. When Mala came into the room, he told us that he found the polyps and that I would need a CT scan and a TURBT (transurethral resection of the bladder tumor). So we go busy making plans for a CT scan on Friday and out-patient surgery one week from Friday.

The combination of Mala's infection and the dense material I saw in my urine had led me to prepare for something like this. I had resumed my imagery and mindfulness practices around a healthy bladder, so I didn't take it too badly.

When we got home, I started down the road of research on bladder polyps and called Michael Broffman. Michael was encouraging and said that in his experience, the polyps are usually benign. We'll see!

## 4/29/10: A Raven or a Hawk?

About a month ago, Mala and I attended a pep talk for the benefit of the Foundation for Shamanic Studies at a beautiful home in Tiburon. Dr. Michael Harner was the featured presenter. I had met him in conjunction with the Institute for Health and Healing event in 2009, where he was honored with the Pioneering Award in Integrative Medicine. He is a lovely man with a warm heart and a peaceful spirit. He is the father of shamanic studies in the whole Western world. Trained as an anthropologist, he spent time in the rain forests of South America studying indigenous cultures and was soon trained in the practices of shamanism. His many books and public talks have made shamanism an acceptable form of integrative medicine.

Susan Mokelke, the foundation director, then spoke about current activities and showed two video clips. One had to do with South American shamans and the other with shamans in Nepalese or Tibetan extract. Then she offered to conduct an evening experience in the practices of shamanism sometime in April, and tonight was the night!

After a short introduction, we did a practice drumming followed by a traditional shamanic journey. We were given the instructions to lie down and cover our eyes to make the room as dark as possible. We were then to descend to the "lower world" through some chosen mechanism and greet an animal. From there, we should just observe or experience.

Susan kept the drum beat for 15 minutes. I started at the top of the stairs leading down to China Cove in Point Lobos State Reserve near Carmel, California. There are 101 steps leading to the beach, but I seemed to float down them at a remarkable pace. Once at the bottom of the stairs, I crossed the beach and slid under the green seaweed that always accumulates there. Within an instant, I was transported to the so-called lower world, where I found myself on a deck of a cabin located about half way down into a forest valley. I lay on the deck and a large bird – either a raven or a hawk. Almost instantaneously after the bird arrived, it started pecking away at the polyps. Frequently, it would leave, possibly to feed little ones, but it continued to come back to peck away until the returning beats were sounded on the drum.

When I shared the experience with my partner in the journey I recognized the possibility that the bird, which also may have been a falcon, may have pecked away both polyps completely. This would not be the first time that I have seen masses disappear. When Micah was nine, he was rushed to the hospital with a stomach ache which turned out to appear to be a mass in his abdomen based on x-ray data. Mala and I rushed back to the hospital to be with him and the next pictures revealed no such mass. We were there to provide love and support and a whole lot more.

**4/30/10: CT Scan**

Today, I had an uneventful CT scan as planned. I won't know the results until May 12.

**5/2/10: Lunch at the Club**

Dr. Martin Rossman met me at the Harbor Point Tennis and Swim Club for a long delayed birthday lunch (his). The club was crowded with swimmers, tennis players, and spectators, so it took an hour to get our food! But it was a beautiful, warm day and Harbor Point is not a bad place to be. I chose this spot because I had arranged to play in the late morning.

I shared my experience of the shamanic journey with him in as much detail as possible. I knew that from his vast knowledge and experience with guided imagery that he would not offer an opinion of the journey, but he did think that it represents a "good omen."

I joined TeamInspire tonight. I'd like to invite other members to check out this site and Mindfulness in Healing. Please check out my profile.

**5/3/2010: Pre-op Exam**

I had an appointment today with Dr. Nagar in Sausalito. She is a young woman (compared to me!) with a lot of knowledge and enthusiasm who speaks very rapidly which is typical of Indians. I like her a lot. She had a hard time believing that I was 70! My exam was mostly uneventful and included an EKG, but I have to give more blood tests tomorrow for determination of liver function, thyroid, and other conditions not measured by Dr. Neuwirth's tests. No big deal! I'll go tomorrow at 8:00 and it will be done with.

**5/5/2010: News of the Day**

I received three new pieces of information today that are worthy of reporting:

The blood tests from yesterday revealed that my TSH was slightly high.

I shouldn't play tennis for a week after the surgery - boo!

The CT scan revealed no spread of disease - this is good news!

In addition, my boss was very forgiving of my situation.

Check out this link on Extra about a cancer cure in Los Angeles by Dr. Paul Song. I believe that El Camino Hospital in Mountain View, CA has the same device as Dr. Song.

## 5/6/2010: Surgery Tomorrow

This evening was the final lecture in the IHH mini-medical series on The Brain Revealed – From Chemistry to Mystery. I knew that Dr. Molly Roberts was speaking, so in spite of surgery scheduled for tomorrow, Mala and I went to hear her talk and Carolyn met us there. It was phenomenal! She spoke on the connection between the brain, five senses, and integrative medicine. You can probably get her slides early next week from the IHH web site. I was extremely moved by her talk, as I actually am involved in many of the activities she recommended.

Another wonderful thing happened: Sandra Harner brought me a CD on Shamanic Drumming from the Foundation for Shamanic Studies, which was founded by her husband, Dr. Michael Harner. I felt really blessed that she would make such a genuine offer of generosity to me.

All of this had the effect of increasing my state of calm for the surgery tomorrow.

## 5/7/10: TURBT

The surgery went well, at least as far as the reports I've received so far have shown. I lingered in the recovery room until about 10:15. I wanted to be sure that I would have minimal problems with the after effects of the anesthesia, so I stayed a little longer than expected. I was fed some juice and crackers and that seemed to satisfy me for a while.

At home, Mala has made chicken soup and a baked potato for lunch. I spend most of the day going in and out of sleep and watching the blood flow out of my bladder. I spent much time meditating and watching Stephen Hawking's series on Into the Universe from the Discovery Channel. Night came quickly, but sleep was a little difficult until I took my regular doses of melatonin, Bone Up and D3. I had to use the bathroom about five times during the night, but managed to get a good night's sleep.

## 5/8/2010: At Home

Today, the bleeding was less and by the early evening, it stopped.

My girls came by for lunch and Carolyn came over as they were leaving. Having company helped me keep my mind off of my bladder. My main concern is still how to prevent further polyps.

## 5/9/2010: Mother's Day

I spent the morning doing research on new developments in bladder cancer. I visited the Bladder Cancer Advocacy Network and watched some videos from the November, 2009 Patient Forum. The information was kind of distressing. At the same time KGO TV had a special on new developments in cancer and one of the segments was on bladder cancer. Obviously, this was the most interesting segment for me and you can watch it too.

Mother's day was really nice. The girls made smoke salmon pizza and chocolate covered strawberries which were yummy! The Rossmans shared the meal and the day with us until late in the afternoon.

## 5/12/2010: Less Good News

I had my meeting with Dr. Neuwirth this afternoon. The news was not that good. The two polyps were actual T1 tumors, which he removed during the TURBT last week. The good news is that BCG treatments should be quite effective against further tumors. The bad news is that it is my bladder that has to undergo these treatments. Dr. Neuwirth seemed hopeful, however. I start the BCG treatments in two weeks and I have to go once a week for six weeks.

BCG (Bacillus Calmette-Guerin) is a bacterial preparation of a strain of tuberculosis vaccine. It is instilled in the bladder with a catheter and needs to remain there at least two hours. The last instillation in 1998 lasted 12 years. So if this works as well as the list time, I'll be 82!

I felt like I had just lost an important tennis match – kind of down and low energy. Fortunately, Lady Catherine (my daughter's best friend) came for dinner and took a lot of the sting out of the news. After she left, I spoke with Mala and the girls and could feel their love and concern. Their reaction was surprisingly calm, as they have a lot of love for me and know that my mindfulness practices and integrative medicine with get me through.

## 5/14/2010: Appointment with Michael Broffman

My appointment with Michael Broffman at the Pine Street Clinic took place this afternoon for about two-and-one-half hours.

It's all about aging. Bladder cancer is a disease in older men (and women). More about this later.

Michael said that I needed about 50 grams protein/day with about 2 quarts of water, a minimum of 1000 calories, and a low carbohydrate intake. Some of the protein can be gotten from rice or whey powders. This amounts to about .78 grams/kilo of protein. In connection with protein, he mentioned the research of Otto Warburg and Brian Peskin. Warburg got a Nobel Prize for demonstrating that oxygen deprived cells develops cancer. I asked about hyperbaric oxygen therapy and he said that it would be good for this reason.

I asked about what other treatments he would recommend and he gave me three ideas. The first is a substance called Gc-MAF. There is a Google video, which explains, "Gc-MAF triggers our immune response to cancer. Cancer cells deactivate Gc-MAF. Dr. Nobuto Yamamoto has shown that laboratory preparation and injections of Gc-MAF bypasses the cancer's deactivation process and allows the macrophages to attack. This procedure has resulted in 100 percent cure rates for 4 to 7 years, the length of the studies to date. There are no side effects." Michael said that you had to inject the Gc-MAF to be effective.

The second product in Michael's bag of tricks is DCA or dichloroacetate. According to the DCA site, DCA "worked to reactivate the apoptosis mechanism of cancer cells, causing rapid shrinkage of tumors in rats. Mitochondrial reactivation represents an entirely new approach to treating cancer." He recommended taking this during BCG treatments plus about 6 months. The dosage of 500mg corresponds to about 1/8 teaspoon and 100g should last me through the whole treatment. Sodium dichloroacetate can be purchased in Canada, but not in the US.

The third product is resveratrol. According to Life Extension,

"Findings from published scientific literature indicate that resveratrol may be the most effective plant extract for maintaining optimal health and promoting longevity." I've known about this for a while and almost ordered it several months ago, but I failed to do so.

Michael recommended several products to try post BCG treatments. These include pomegranate, curcumin and green tea extracts.

The anti-ageing plan begins after BCG with a 24 hour urine test for hormones and their metabolites. The goal is to bring testosterone up to the level of a 35 year old man. There will be herb supplements to support hormone replenishment. Another hormone of interest is aldosterone. A constitutional homeopathic remedy may also be used in this project.

New cancer treatments include HIFU in China. This stands for high intensity focused ultrasound and may now be available in the US.

I spoke about two other conditions that concern me. The first was acid reflux when I have too much food or lots of garlic and onions. Michael told me that the active ingredient in Tagamet, cimetidine is not only good to relive acid indigestion, but it has some immune and cancer fighting qualities. So I guess it is not too bad to rely on this when conditions dictate it.

My sleep problem could be helped by time-release melatonin. He said the blue or red lights don't upset melatonin metabolism.

Both Mala and I felt really encouraged by this session. It seems like the BCG treatment is just a bump in the road and I should be cancer free when it is complete.

## 05/18/2010: Hyperbaric Oxygen Therapy

Thirteen years ago, Michael Broffman told me about hyperbaric oxygen therapy. At that time, it was available in Europe, but now it is available locally. I had previously experienced a session with Dr. Geoffry Saft of Hyperbaric Oxygen Therapy in Larkspur, CA. Now I am getting treatments in preparation for BCG.

Today's experience was quite wonderful. I was relaxed and probably slept a bit. The rest of the time I listened to Jon Kabat-Zinn, founder of Mindfulness Based Stress Reduction at the University of Massachusetts. I'll probably have a treatment every day until the BCG treatments start, and maybe until they end!

Hyperbaric oxygen therapy works by sending oxygen under pressure into the blood stream. The research of Dr. Otto Warburg had proved that oxygen starved cells are more likely to develop cancer than those which have plenty of oxygen. So the theory is that oxygen at higher than atmospheric pressures can facilitate blood flow to the cells.

**5/20/2010: Tennis!**

I had my second hyperbaric oxygen therapy today, and it was similar to the first. I was hoping that it would propel me through an hour and a half of tennis without any problems, but I was exhausted after about one hour. I started missing badly after that and had to take a nap before Mindfulness in Healing. By the way, the Mindfulness in Healing Well-being Support group is moving to Tuesday evenings from 7:30 to 9:00 at the Pine Street Clinic.

# EPILOG

Now that you have completed reading ***Stop Cancer in its Tracks: Your Path to Mindfulness in Healing Yourself***, please consider doing what you can to help people who are suffering. Many people can be relieved of certain types of suffering by following a daily routing of mindfulness meditation, exercise, and self-compassion.

Almost immediately after my first glimpse of being cancer free (which was not true) I felt like I had something to give back to my community in some form other than my daily posts on my website. I played around with the name *Mindfulness and ART in Healing* for a while and even was invited to teach a sample class in late July of 1997. The class was a success and this was as far as it went at that time in my life.

Between 1998 and 2004, I bought my first house, lost my job, found another, cleaned up a significant mudslide at our house, lost my job again, started an internet business with a friend, and was hired by the Technical Committee (TC) of the Department of Justice (DoJ) to monitor Microsoft's compliance with the settlement agreement. In the first two months of this assignment, I discovered documentation errors that triggered a massive effort by the TC and the DoJ to hire 50 more engineers to monitor Microsoft. I was able to get jobs for many of my friends and this brought me a lot of joy.

We would get together about once a week to discuss technical issues and I was extremely happy with the progress we made and the benefits of working on a team.

As we smoothly established our rhythm, I began to look for ways to give back to my community again. This led me to serve on the Board of Directors of the Marin AIDS Project and the Community Council of the Institute for Health and Healing concurrently between 2007 and 2010. These opportunities to participate in the greater good of my community inspired me to develop my own program.

Thus, on the Summer solstice of 2009, I held the first <u>Mindfulness in Healing</u> group at the Pine Street Clinic in San Anselmo, California on Wednesday nights. We had been gathering there to meditate on a regular basis for about a year as a *sangha* (spiritual community) for about a year. Our sangha was formed in 2001 and interest in it faded in early 2009, so I took the opportunity to start the group.

The principles of *Mindfulness in Healing* are derived from the teachings of mindfulness applied to health and healing. Together with my partner, Carolyn DeFay, L. C. S. W. we offer a safe space for people to come and share with us about what is going on in their lives.

Compassionate listening and loving speech are the foundations of our sharing practice. As mindfulness deepens awareness of our experience we find new ways to enhance our own well-being. We become able to transform our suffering and find freedom in the present moment, embracing a feeling of wellness.

We offer guided meditation and relaxation exercises to help promote a calm, clear mind and a peaceful, loving heart. This energy supports us in accepting our challenges just as they are and leads to increased well-being and wellness.

I discovered that I have a knack for feeling what is going on in the group and spontaneously offer a valuable guided meditation that everyone enjoys. This has been the most wonderful take away from the almost four years (as I write this in May, 2013) of holding *Mindfulness in Healing*.

It is with great joy that either Carolyn or myself and most often, both of us open the doors of the Pine Street Clinic to all who want to come. Our drop-in format is flexible and works very well. You are welcome to join in whenever you are in the neighborhood.

For more information about *Mindfulness in Healing*, please visit http://mindfulnessinhealing.org.

If you register your copy of *Stop Cancer In Its Tracks: How to Embrace Mindfulness in Healing* at http://mindfulnessinhealing.org/register-stop-cancer, you will be able to follow the healing progress through the **Stop Cancer** on the menu bar. Certain new materials may be password protected, and registering will reveal the password to you and qualify you to see the password protect materials.

## PARTING WORDS

In the Buddhist tradition, we have a practice of sharing the merit of whatever we do. In this case, I offer the following verses:

> *May the merit of my suffering and recovery benefit all beings and bring peace.*
> *May you be save from internal and external harm.*
> *May you have a calm, clear mind and a peaceful, loving heart.*
> *May you be strong, healthy, and vital.*
> *May you experience love, joy, wonder, and wisdom in this life, just as it is.*
> *May all beings be happy, truly happy.*

## ABOUT THE AUTHOR

Dr. Jerome Freedman is an author, healthcare advocate, mindfulness meditation teacher, and a cancer survivor since 1997. He is a long-time practitioner in the tradition of Zen Master Thich Nhat Hanh in which he is an ordained member of the Order of Interbeing. His recent article in The Mindfulness Bell titled "Healthy and Free" touched many people. He is also a certified teacher of the Enneagram in the Oral Tradition with Helen Palmer.

Jerome currently teaches **Mindfulness in Healing** at the Pine Street Clinic in San Anselmo, California and writes daily on his blog, **Meditation Practices**. He is a contributing author of *I Am With You: Love Letters to Cancer Patients*, Nancy Novak, PhD, and Barbara K. Richardson.

Dr. Freedman served on Board of Directors of the Marin AIDS Project and the Advisory Council of the Institute for Health and Healing between 2007 and 2010. He is now a major contributor to the Buddhist Climate Action Network and the Earth Holder Sangha – the Plum Village climate response community - as an activist promoting earth protection. He is also a technical advisor for Operation Diana, an NGO dedicated to the survival of elephants in Africa.

Dr. Freedman holds a Ph. D. in computer science, along with two master's degrees in physics and a bachelor's degree in chemical engineering. He still consults internationally on software engineering problems and expert witness cases. He successfully interviewed Dr. Neil deGrasse Tyson on cosmology and Buddhist thought in 2011.

He can be reached by for consultations, dharma talks, lectures, and days of mindfulness by email at jerome [at] mountainsangha [dot] org.

*Also by Dr. Freedman*

*Mindfulness Breaks: Your Path to Awakening*

*Stop Cancer in its Tracks: Your Path to Mindfulness in Healing Yourself*

*Healing Cancer with Your Mind: 7 Strategies to Help YOU Survive*

*Seven Steps to Stop Interruptions in Meditation: How to Concentrate and*

*Focus on Your Meditation and Deal with Distractions*

*Cosmology and Buddhist Thought: A Conversation with Dr. Neil deGrasse Tyson – excerpted by Lion's Roar Buddhist Magazine*

*The Enneagram: Know Your Type! Awaken Your Potential!*

*Contributing author* to *I Am With You: Love Letters to Cancer Patients*[i] published February, 2015.

Mindfulness Break Recordings

Anger Control Mindfulness Break
Achieve Goals Mindfulness Break
Sound Sleep Mindfulness Break
Stress Relief Mindfulness Break
Reduce Symptoms Mindfulness Break
Weight Loss Mindfulness Break

    Order from [mountainsangha.org/products](mountainsangha.org/products).

**DEDICATION**

This book is dedicated to my family –
    Mala, my wife of more than 30 years
    My son Micah
    My daughters Rachael and Jessica
    And
    To all the many practitioners who helped me along the path to recovery.

## ACKNOWLEDGEMENTS

First and foremost I want to thank my family for their continued support throughout my healing experience.

My wife, Mala, was always there for me – through pain and sorrow. She went to every appointment and held my hand during the infusion of chemotherapy cocktails. She brought me food and drink when I couldn't get out of bed. She helped me limp around after the surgery on my thigh and shoulder. I don't know what I would have done without her.

Then I want to thank my children, Micah, Rachael, and Jessica. The children were always around and they did not seem too worried. In June, 1997, Rachael graduated from Marin Horizon School to go on to high school. I remember how much I cried during the speech she gave.

Then I must thank my healers.

Michael Broffman served as my guide and quarterback through conventional and alternative treatments. I am really grateful for all he has done to help save my bladder and recover from cancer.

Dr. Martin Rossman was a true friend and splendid healer for me. He attended my meeting with Dr. Neuwirth when he announced my diagnosis.

Dr. Sara Huang was actually the person who may have had the most significant impact on saving my bladder. She is a longtime family friend and head radiation oncologist at a major San Francisco hospital. Sara connected me with Dr. William U. Shipley, whose bladder sparing protocol played a major role in my treatment.

Leslie Davenport provided psychological support for Mala and me during the whole ordeal. Her work with me with interactive guided imagery and other techniques allowed me to find some inner resources to facilitate resilience and insight. You'll see what I mean when you read the section from the spring equinox of 1997.

My team of doctors, Dr. Harry Neuwirth (urologist), Dr. David Gullion (oncologist), Dr. Francine Halberg (radiation oncologist), and Dr. Robert Belknap (family doctor) were all wonderfully supportive and helpful during my crisis months. To my surprise, they all cooperated in administering the Shipley bladder sparing protocol and I am eternally grateful for their efforts.

There are many other people that deserve a huge round of applause for their contributions to my well-being. Most, if not all, are mentioned in the pages that follow. Please do not underestimate their importance in my healing experience.

www.ingramcontent.com/pod-product-compliance
Lightning Source LLC
LaVergne TN
LVHW021714060526
838200LV00050B/2663